Praise for **Your Persona**

"If you have challenges with food, weight, and yo-yo dieting, this book is for you! *Your Personal Journey with Food* is thought-provoking, challenges you to look deep within yourself, understand your behavior regarding food, and how to undo unhealthy attachments.

Tracy and Ingrid are such amazing health coaches. It literally feels like they are right there with you, personally coaching you!

Your Personal Journey with Food helps you;
* Examine all aspects of life that are contributing factors to how you are living and want to live your life.
* How those factors are affecting your overall health, and how to make small changes to improve.
* Slow down and be mindful, eat with intention, and pay attention to what is happening in your body.

Your Personal Journey with Food gives you;
This book gives you the tools to:
* Set yourself up for success daily and deal with challenges or situations.
* Guidance on other foundational aspects such as exercise, daily water intake, sleep, stress management, and how to be healthy mentally and physically.
* The authors are fantastic in their delivery of how to navigate delicate issues and how to have more self-respect.

I love that there are spaces to make notes, write thoughts, and answer questions while working through the journey.

I highly recommend this book to anyone wanting to understand their relationships with food, understand their behavior with food, and make a change in their lives for the better."

–Dr. Teresa Richter, http://www.kirklandnaturalmedicine.com/

"There are so many people who suffer from eating disorders and obesity. Tracy and Ingrid have done a great job walking the reader along a personal journey to understanding their relationship with food, which is key to successful weight management. With all the potential health risks being obese presents, I absolutely see a need for this book."

–Jenifer Bunge, Certified Personal Trainer, Certified Cancer Exercise Specialist

"Tracy and Ingrid, thank you for opening your hearts in this book. Tracy and Ingrid are so eloquent and complement each other through the entire book. I am inspired to wake up and do better. To look in the mirror and be honest with me.

The wisdom and love are not only expressed but felt with each word read. I thought I was a Master at making mindful choices, but Ingrid and Tracy invited me to see past my fears and look in the rearview mirror. Bringing forward old wounds with food, I had forgotten I had and needed to heal from. This is a step by step guide, an invitation to take your control back, to relearn the basics and beyond. I love the integration of whole-body wellness. Seeing the entire body-mind-spirit aspects and anchoring them into everyday choices. Beautiful, inspiring work. I am ready to create a love for food and my body again. Thank you."

–Chastity Kribble, Author, LMT, Multi-Dimensional Healer
at www.theartofmetta.com

"A thoughtful, precise, and very personal book, *Your Personal Journey With Food* is jam-packed with value for any person wanting to understand themselves and their relationship with their own body. I love how interactive it is; it's really like having your own personal health coach in your own two hands!"

–Lisa Ann Williams, M.A. CEO of StoryShift, www.LisaAnnWilliams.com

"I loved this book by Ingrid Lauw and Tracy Schroeder-Cromwell. The approach to *Your Personal journey with Food* by Ingrid and Tracy feels non-judgmental and full of joy. The holistic approach and road maps, journals, and exercises create an easy step by step total health plan."

–Karen Rae, Owner and Founder of Fave Lifestyles www.favelifestyles.com

"The name of this book is spot on! *Your Personal Journey with Food* is full of helpful, straightforward tips and methods to assist in identifying, facilitating, and ultimately creating accountability without being too rigid. The authors have put in the work and it shows! This beautiful book is going to be hugely helpful to so many people as it makes its way into the hearts and hands of many."

–Brenda Baker, Certified Integrative Nutrition Health Coach, Author of *Oddly Colorful* and *Tendra the Turkey* https://amzn.to/32z9Lg6

"Yet again, Tracy & Ingrid hit it out of the park!!! Another homerun! If you ever doubt if this book is right for you, or if Tracy or Ingrid are the right people to support you with your relationship with food, let me say this: GET THIS BOOK BECAUSE THEY KNOW THEIR STUFF! You may think: "Yet another 'losing weight' book in the already large library of weight management?" Well, let me tell you, this one is different. Different in the sense that Tracy and Ingrid are only mentioning "the outcome" while powerfully dealing with "the cause" of being overweight and having a troubling relationship with food. Because let's face it, being overweight is a result of a deeper issue that almost never is about the food itself but has everything to do with THE RELATIONSHIP you have with food. In this book, Tracy and Ingrid present you with powerful exercises. These exercises will, when you do them, change your entire relationship with food and your body. So, let me reiterate the "when you do them" part. Because all too often, we skip over that and then say it didn't work. This book was written for you. Change your relationship with food, your body and your mind, and your life will change in ways you can't even imagine. To your health and happiness,"

–Jacob Melaard, Life and Relationship Coach, Master NLP practitioner, Strategic Intervention Coach

"I didn't know much about the lymphatic system until cancerous cells were found in my lymph nodes. Talk about not knowing what you have until it's gone! With 14 lymph nodes removed with the mastectomy, I am much more familiar with the support my lymphatic system needs from me. I wish I had this book at that point.

Ingrid and Tracy have given you a chance to look at your body in terms of the support, the love, care, and attention it needs so you can appreciate it. "Your Personal Journey with Food" is full of important information, solid tips, and straight-up advice all broken down so we can move beyond frustration and embark on a journey with clarity."

"This book is one of a kind! I've been working with health and nutrition the past 20 years but this book gave me so much insight and I learned so much in such a short amount of time. This book REALLY covers all you need to know on HOW everything is connected and affecting your overall health and Well-being. This book will truly take you on your own personal journey, like no other book you've ever read!"

YOUR PERSONAL
JOURNEY
WITH FOOD

YOUR PERSONAL JOURNEY WITH FOOD

A ROADMAP FOR THE CONFUSED AND FRUSTRATED DIETER

INGRID LAUW &
TRACY SCHROEDER-CROMWELL

Tanzanite Books

The materials in this book is not meant to replace a doctor's care. It is not meant to give a diagnosis or promise to cure, heal, or reverse a diagnosis. The authors are only offering information of general nature that may be part of a journey for well-being. THE READER SHOULD CONSULT WITH THEIR OWN PERSONAL DOCTOR PRIOR TO INTEGRATING ANY OF THE PROTOCOLS DISCUSSED IN THIS BOOK AND THE AUTHORS AND PUBLISHER ASSUME NO RESPONSIBILITY FOR THE DIRECT OR INDIRECT CONSEQUENCES OF FOLLOWING SUCH PROTOCOLS.

The author and publisher are providing this book and its contents on an "as is" basis and make no representations or warranties of any kind with respect to this book or its contents. THE AUTHOR AND PUBLISHER DISCLAIMM ALL REPRESENTATIONS AND WARRANTIES INCLUDING, BUT NOT LIMITED TO WARRANTIES OF MERCHANTABILITY AND HEALTHCARE FOR A PARTICULAR PURPOSE. In addition, the author and publisher do not represent or warrant that the information accessible via this book is accurate, complete or current. The statements made about products and services have not been evaluated by the U.S. Food and Drug Administration. They are not intended to diagnose, treat, cure, or prevent any condition or disease.

ISBN: 978-1-7350516-1-1 (Paperback)
ISBN: 978-1-7350516-0-4 (ebook)

Library of Congress Control Number: 2020908766

Editing by: Judith Carrell
Cover design by: Max Rosales
Interior design by: Constellation Book Services

Printed in the United States of America.

First printing edition 2020.

Published and distributed by: Tanzanite Books, LLC, www.journeywithfood.com

DEDICATION

We dedicate this book to all of our readers.

We are excited to not only share our Personal Journey with Food with you but walk alongside you as you travel yours.

Everyone's journey is different. We are all unique beings, and we all have our own life stories. Thus, we are all where we are for various reasons. As you enter into these pages, we hope that you will embrace the journey that has brought you to where you are today and then embrace the road you are about to travel.

Know that you are worthy. You are worthy of this next journey. You are worthy of self-care and self-love.

Welcome to Your Personal Journey with Food.

Ingrid and Tracy

Contents

I Think I'm Lost!
Where's the Search
and Rescue Team?

Congratulations!

Congratulations for choosing to invest in yourself.

You are about to set off on a journey in which you will be creating a relationship with food that serves you in a healthy and supportive way. This journey is going to be an exciting time for you, as well as a challenging one.

We don't want to mislead you and tell you that the journey will not be without doubt, moments of sadness, and moments of uncertainty. It will. We can tell you that *Your Personal Journey with Food* will be one that creates strength, understanding, awareness, and healthy change.

The goal of this book is to get you started on your own *Personal Journey with Food*. It will take you on a path of self-discovery in which you will get a better understanding of why you may be lost regarding what foods are right for you and why you are making and have made certain food choices in the past.

On this journey, you will also take steps that will begin moving you forward. Forward into YOUR future, leading you to a healthy relationship with food.

Are you uncertain as to where you are? Are you lost and looking for help regarding what foods work best for your body? Figuring all of this out can be a real challenge.

By the time you finish reading this book, complete all the exercises, and put them into ACTION, you will know where you are. You will also be implementing the personalized steps and actions necessary to get you to your desired relationship with food. Now, notice we did not say after you finish reading this book. We said, by the time you finish reading this book AND complete all the exercises AND take action. As with any book or program, if you just read it and don't take any ACTION, nothing will change. We invite you to participate and fully commit. By doing so, you will discover what you need to do to change your life regarding your food. By fully participating, you will build the strength necessary to implement those changes.

You purchased this book for a reason. Commit the time you need to read, complete the exercises, and embrace *Your Personal Journey with Food* as it begins to unfold in front of you. Embrace it in all its messiness and beauty. We understand that there may be a part of you that is afraid of change. Afraid of what you may discover. You may be fearful that since you have tried so many diets and other programs that this book won't help you. Just remember, everything you have experienced in the past has been a learning experience. It has prepared you for this book. All you need to do is commit to taking each step that we ask you to.

Commit to you. You deserve a healthy relationship with food. You deserve to feel good in your body. You deserve to be healthy. You deserve loving and rewarding relationships. You deserve a fulfilling relationship with yourself, filled with self-love and respect.

Let's figure out where you are. When you are lost and cannot figure out where you are, how do you get where you want to go? Getting lost doesn't relate only to where you are physically on the earth; you can get lost inside your own body, lost inside your mind. Uncertain of where to turn. Unsure of what is right for you.

We were both lost as well. We were unsure as to how we got where we were with our health. We didn't know how our relationship with food got out of hand and sent us in the wrong direction. Eventually, through trial and error, we did find our own personal paths and now have healthy relationships with food. We are honored to walk with you as you find yours.

When you get lost, there are several things you can do.

1. At the moment you realize you are lost, stop and wait for the search and rescue team to find you.
2. Retrace your steps and start your journey over with hopes that you are going to take the correct route next time you progress.
3. Ask for help from someone who knows the way.
4. Utilize a map or GPS.
5. Give up and aimlessly wander, hoping you will figure out where you are.

In this book, you will be utilizing steps one through four.

To get started, you will be taking an assessment. This assessment is step one, as listed above. You are stopping and waiting for the search and rescue team to find you. Answer the assessment questions honestly. If you choose not to, the rescue team, which has headed out to find you, will have a challenging time doing so.

It will be a bit scary for the search and rescue team, as the path is not smooth and easy. It's a bit bumpy, winding, with a lot of curves and hills. There may even be things along this path that scare the search and rescue team. So much so, they may want to quit. They may turn away for a moment. But they are committed, and they will keep looking for you. They won't give up!

Would you like to know something empowering? YOU are the leader of the search and rescue team! You, along with the following questionnaire, and this book, are going to find out where you are! This is very powerful!

When someone gets lost, they can feel as if they are a big failure. Remember, it is not a sentence of failure. People get lost and in many ways. With this in mind, the assessment is not a reason to take out your mental whip and give yourself 50 lashes. Yes, we can attest that the truth as to where you are might be scary to see, but please believe us when we tell you that until you are honest with where you are, it is difficult to take the correct steps to find your way to your healthy relationship with food. (When Tracy first assessed herself, she got a horrible feeling in the pit of her stomach. It was hard to see the reality of where she was. She now embraces that moment because she finally accepted who she was. She took responsibility for what got her to where she was. She was ready to embrace her journey, her life, and her relationship with food for the better.)

We Forget to Look Under the Hood

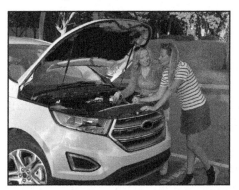

Think of it this way, when you prepare to take your car on a long road trip, you assess its mechanical ability to make the journey successfully. In the assessment of your vehicle, you or a mechanic will look under the hood, check engine fluid levels, check any important belts, timing chains, etc. The mechanic would also look at the brakes and possibly rotate the tires. If something requires repair, you would have the repair done and then be on your way. As humans, we tend not to look at our lives or our bodies this way. We may put the wrong fuel into our body, causing it to run rough. Just as a car needs the right fuel to run, so does your body.

Let's take a look under the hood. Below is a circle that we call your "Life Radar." Please rate each of the areas of the radar on a scale of 1 to 5. 1 meaning you feel least accomplished or satisfied in this area to 5 being you feel very confident and satisfied in this area. After plotting your answers, connect the dots so that you can see how your radar looks. Note the date you complete this exercise, as this date will be significant as you travel your journey.

Life Radar

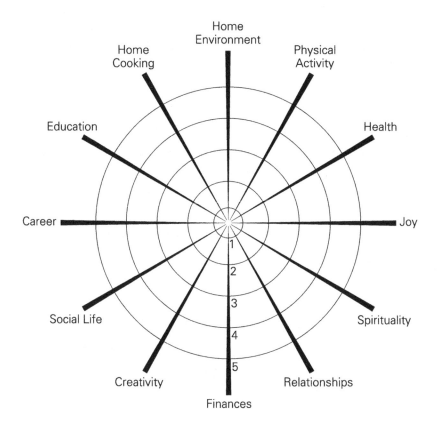

Wait a minute! Ingrid and Tracy, I only see two items on this radar that possibly relate to food? Health and Home Cooking? What could any of the other areas on the list have to do with food?

Our answer, "Absolutely EVERYTHING!" Our lives are connected—every aspect.

Let's look at it like this. You go to get your car looked at before your long road trip. Although you were giving it the proper fuel for its engine, some of the parts are wearing out and causing stress to the vehicle and engine. You also find that your tires are worn and need replacing. These repairs have nothing to do with the fuel you put into your car, but they have everything to do with your vehicle's ability to run efficiently and safely. Think of all the other items on the list as the integral parts of your life that directly affect how you feel and function, areas that could be affecting your relationship with food. As you work through this book, you will uncover and begin to understand how all of these areas relate to your food and the choices you make around food.

How to Use This Guide

This book is a map that will allow you to explore food and healthy habits to improve your health. We wanted to create a map that will assist both the beginner and the expert explorer.

This map has three parts:

- ⊕ Departure area (chapters 1 to 4): information to help you start your journey
- ⊕ Exploration area (chapters 5 to 14): your personalized path
- ⊕ Reflection area (chapter 15): your opportunity to revisit what you have learned and move forward with new confidence

The first four chapters are the "departure" area, and this is why we recommend that you read these chapters in order.

Chapters 5 to 14 are your specific *"Personal Journey."* Utilize the questionnaire on the following pages to establish YOUR PERSONALIZED order in which to read these chapters. With that said, feel free to read these chapters in any order your inner self believes is right for you.

We hope that you see your answers as valuable information to help you move forward on *Your Personal Journey with Food*. Your responses are neither good nor bad. They are just your answers—only information to help you find your starting point.

Feet on the Pavement View

Put today's date above the first column, then rate your answers on a scale of 1 to 5. One being least like you to, 5 is most like you. Do this for each section.

Chapter 5—Time for an Alignment

THE PATH OF MINDFULNESS

Date		
I eat at the table when I am at home.		
I am ok leaving food on my plate if I am full.		
I don't eat at my desk.		
I pay attention to my food when eating.		
I always put my eating utensils down between each bite.		
I always chew each bite of food at least 15-20 times before swallowing.		
I know how food affects me physically and emotionally.		
I know when I am full.		
Total		

Chapter 6 – Your Journey Buddies

SYMPTOMS AS A CO-PILOT

Date		
I have not been diagnosed with any of the following medical conditions. (If you have, please circle each one that pertains to you. If you have another diagnosis that is not listed, please add it to the list.)		

Autoimmune Diseases

Alopecia Areata
Antiphospholipid Syndrome
Autoimmune Hepatitis
Celiac Disease
Chron's Disease
Chronic Fatigue Syndrome
Dermatomyositis
Grave's Disease
Guillain-Barré Syndrome
Hashimoto's Thyroiditis
Inflammatory Bowel Disease
Multiple Sclerosis
Myasthenia Gravis
Pernicious Anemia
Primary Biliary Cirrhosis
Psoriasis
Psoriatic Arthritis
Rheumatoid Arthritis
Sarcoidosis
Systemic Scleroderma
Sjögren's Syndrome
Systemic Lupus Erythematosus
Type 1 Diabetes
Ulcerative Colitis
Vitiligo

Common Diseases

Alzheimer's
Arteriosclerosis
Breast Cancer
Colon Cancer
Chronic Liver Disease/Cirrhosis
Chronic Obstructive Pulmonary
    Disease – COPD
Type 2 Diabetes
Hypertension
Heart Disease – Ischaemic,
    Congenital
Nephritis/CRF
Obesity
Peripheral Arterial Disease
Prostate Cancer
Stroke

Date		
I don't have any of the following symptoms. (If you do have symptoms, please circle each one that pertains to you. If you have another symptom not listed, please write it down here as well.)		

Acid reflux
Acne
Appetite – low to none
Arthritis
Bags under the eyes
Bloating
Bloody stools
Brain fog
Constipation
Colds - frequent
Cravings
Dark circles under the eyes
Depression
Diarrhea
Digestion – painful
Dizziness
Dry eyes
Eczema
Edema, such as swelling of the
   hands, ankles, feet
Fatigue
Fever – chronic
Gas
Gums – swollen and bleeding
Hair loss
Hives
Headaches/migraines
Heartburn
Heart – rapid rate (arrhythmia)
Hearing loss/ringing in the ear

High cholesterol
Hormonal disorder
Hunger - constant
Insulin resistance
Itchy anus
Itchy mouth or ear canal
Itchy skin
Joint pain
Joint stiffness
Joint swelling
Mood – low
Mood – short-tempered, anger
   and frustration
Muscle spasms, cramps
Nasal Congestion
Nausea
Neurological problems
Numbness, tingling, or burning
   hands or feet
Obesity
Overweight
Puffiness
Sinus infections
Sleep – restless
Psoriasis
Painful and/or irregular
   menstruation
Redness of the skin around eyes
Runny Nose
Sleeplessness

Chapter 6 continued

Sleepiness
Sneezing
Stomach Pain – Burning
Stomach Pain – Cramping
Thirst – frequent and excessive
Urination - frequent

Underweight or extreme thinness
Urination – painful
Urination – dark colored
Uterine Contractions
Viruses – frequent
Weak bones

Answer from page 10.		
Answer from page 11.		
My skin is glowing and looks healthy.		
I have limited to no cravings for sugar.		
I don't have anxiety.		
My body is functioning very well.		
I don't take any prescription medications.		
I am at a "healthy" weight for my height.		
Total		

Chapter 7—Picking the Right Fuel

FOOD SENSITIVITIES

Date		
I don't have any of the autoimmune or chronic diseases listed in the Chapter 6 questionnaire.		
I don't have any of the symptoms listed in the Chapter 6 questionnaire.		
I have completed a guided food elimination diet.		
I have had a food sensitivity panel done.		
I know the difference between a food allergy and a food sensitivity.		
I have a clear head and can easily think.		
I don't take any over-the-counter medications for digestive challenges.		
I don't take any prescribed medications for digestive challenges.		
Total		

Chapter 8—Rest Stop

GET UP AND MOVE

Date		
I get 30 minutes of exercise, such as those listed below, at least four times a week. Walking—Running—Cycling—Yoga—Weight Training, Community Sports Program—Cross-fit—Organized Gym Classes—Self-training at Gym—Hiking—Dance—Playing actively with children		
I am very active at my job.		
I am not afraid of exercise.		
I don't have any physical injuries preventing me from exercising.		
I feel strong in my body and am able to live my life actively whenever I want.		
I feel limber and do not have any stiffness in my joints or muscles.		
I have good balance and feel confident when moving my body.		
I don't feel self-conscious when I think about exercising.		
Total		

Chapter 9—Tune-Up

TIME TO DETOX

Date		
I have high energy levels at least 80-90% of the time.		
I eat homemade meals from whole foods, not from a box, at least 80-90% of the time.		
I am able to eat organic food, at least 80-90% of the time.		
I don't eat any processed foods.		
I don't take any prescribed drugs.		
I don't take any over-the-counter medications.		
I am able to think clearly and do not feel "foggy" in the head.		
I don't have any symptoms listed in questions relating to Chapter 6.		
Total		

Chapter 10—An Important Detour

THE CONTROVERSIES OF FOOD

Date		
I know how to read food labels.		
I compare the front label of a food product with the Nutrition Facts as well as the Ingredients list.		
I know how to interpret an ingredients list.		
I understand why grocery stores are set up the way they are.		
I feel confident that I know what real food is.		
I feel confident that the food I purchase is healthy for me.		
I always question the marketing utilized to sell food products.		
I know how I fit into the food industry and the part I play in it.		
Total		

Chapter 11—Emergency!

I'M STUCK AT FULL THROTTLE!—STRESS

Date		
I feel calm inside my body.		
I make sure I take care of me.		
I exercise for 30 minutes at least four times a week.		
I find it easy to stay present mentally, wherever I am.		
Feelings of anxiousness are far and few between.		
I don't clench my teeth.		
I am able to work with others without feeling trapped or losing my temper.		
I am able to openly discuss issues that are upsetting me long before they turn into something big.		
Total		

Chapter 12—Rest Stop

TIME TO GET SOME MUCH-NEEDED SLEEP

Date		
I get 7 to 8 hours of sleep per night at least six nights a week.		
I go to bed at a consistent time every night.		
I don't wake up in the middle of the night, thinking about life and its challenges.		
I wake up rested and ready to go almost every morning.		
My bedroom is set up to allow me to get a good night's sleep.		
I don't have pets or children that wake me in the middle of the night consistently.		
I have a bedtime ritual that allows me to drift off to sleep easily.		
I am confident that my hormones which allow me to sleep at night and rise easily in the morning are at their optimal levels.		
Total		

Chapter 13—Is My Vehicle Good Enough?

SELF-IMAGE

Date		
I feel very comfortable with my body.		
I am not concerned about the way I look.		
I am satisfied with most aspects of my life, such as my spirituality, economic state, food, friendships, relationships, work, health, etc.		
I do not feel that I am less worthy than other people.		
I have a positive relationship with myself.		
I do not try to hide the food I eat from others.		
When I make mistakes, I see it as only a lesson and move on, no bad feelings here.		
I do not try to hide the real me from myself or others.		
Total		

Chapter 14—Respect of Inner Self

Date		
I only have positive dialogs with myself.		
I feel good about the choices I have made for me and respect myself for those choices.		
I am able to say no to invitations that don't serve my health and well-being.		
I honor not only my body but my mind and spirit.		
I never let myself down.		
I am able to move on from mistakes I have made pretty easily. I learn from mistakes and don't harbor them.		
I do what I say I am going to do. I honor my commitments to myself.		
I love myself and my body.		
Total		

What are your thoughts as you look back at all of your answers to the questionnaire? We hope that you see your answers as incredibly valuable information to help you move forward on *Your Personal Journey with Food*. Remember, your answers are neither good nor bad. They are just your answers and only information to help you assess a starting point.

At this time, find the chapter in which you have the lowest assessment score. That will be your chapter 5. Find that chapter on the **Personal Table of Contents** at the end of this chapter. Write the number five in the column "YOU" next to the corresponding chapter. Continue adding your customized chapter order from your lowest assessment score to the highest. If you have a tie between several chapters, trust your gut as to which one you should read first.

For ease of finding your new chapter progressions, we recommend placing a sticky note at the beginning of each chapter with your custom chapter order number on each note. These notes may make it easier on the eyes and brain to go from one to the other if you don't want to keep referencing your customized table of contents.

As you read each chapter, some will include references to free handouts that you can utilize. Be sure to take advantage of these free resources. We have also included a complimentary **Your Personal Journal with Food** journal, as well as a complimentary **Your Personal Journey with Food Journal.** We strongly recommend that you download these two pdf journals at **www.journeywithfood.com** before moving forward with your journey.

Take time with each chapter. Commit to doing the exercises in each chapter. We recommend that you allow one week for each chapter so that you can complete the exercises, apply what you are learning during the week. At the end of each week, complete the mini Your Personal Journal with Food journal located at the end of each chapter.

You will also see that there are some chapters where both Tracy and Ingrid are listed as authors. This means that you will be hearing from both of us in these chapters. In these chapters, the first author speaking will be named first under the chapter name. For example: "By Tracy and Ingrid." In this example, Tracy will be the first one speaking. When the second author begins to speak, you will see her content indented as well as in a different font from the standard text.

OK! It's time to get going. You are now in the driver's seat. It's time to start your journey!

In Health,
Ingrid and Tracy

PLANNING YOUR PERSONAL JOURNEY WITH FOOD

CHAPTER 1

Before You Start Your Journey
By Ingrid

Imagine you are preparing to embark on a marvelous, life-changing trip. I am sure you would do some planning before you left, correct? You would be sure to have everything ready to depart, such as luggage, tickets, money, snacks, and the hotel reservation. If you are driving your car, you will check the gas level, tire pressure, and the brakes to ensure you have a successful journey, one which will take you to the place of your dreams.

Well, your mindset and your body are just like your car. Your mindset can take you to the place you want to be, or it can detour you, taking you far away from your desired destination.

I now invite you to learn how your mindset drives your food choices. To begin your healthy journey with food, you need to know your starting point. In this book, you will explore your thoughts and feelings about the food that you are eating.

Let´s explore some beliefs usually related to food.

Belief 1: Eating Healthy Cannot Be Enjoyable

We all have our favorite foods. We cannot deny that we receive some pleasure in the act of eating. Eating can create joy from newly discovered flavors or the feeling of comfort when we experience a meal from our childhood, our homeland, or our culture.

Have you noticed how many pleasure-related words are used to describe food? Here are some common ones: Enjoyable, Comforting, Appealing, Appetizing, Delectable, Delicious, Delightful, Divine, Enticing, Exquisite, Finger Licking, Heavenly, Lip-Smacking, Luscious, Mouthwatering, Palatable, Pleasant, Pleasing, Satisfying, Scrumptious, Tantalizing, Tasty, and Yummy are just a few.

Science can help explain why we naturally associate food with pleasure. As Daniel Amen, MD (and co-author David Smith, MD,) explain in their book, "Unchain Your Brain," serotonin is the happy, anti-worry and calming neurotransmitter. When serotonin levels in the brain are low, people tend to be worried, rigid, inflexible, anxious, depressed, obsessive, and compulsive. In our diet, we find foods containing the amino acid L-tryptophan, which your body changes into serotonin.

Here are some foods that contain L-tryptophan:

- ⊕ Chocolate
- ⊕ Simple and refined carbohydrates: white bread, pasta, and sugar
- ⊕ Meat
- ⊕ Seafood
- ⊕ Watercress, spirulina, and spinach (This is not a typographical mistake!)

The first four foods in the list above are obviously pleasure-triggering foods. Just think of a Valentine's Day menu: a shrimp pasta entrée, filet mignon, and for dessert, layered chocolate mousse. But for many people, the last bullet on that list of L-tryptophan-containing foods (watercress, spirulina, and spinach) probably doesn't even belong. Watercress is not viewed as a pleasure-triggering food. Some readers might even think there was a printing error.

Why is it surprising to see a food like spinach as a pleasure-inducing food? There is an idea that eating healthy is the opposite of enjoyable. Eating healthy for plenty of people is about dieting, starvation, and restriction. We all know the long list of "bad" foods that you shouldn't taste, smell, or even touch. People that accept this idea as true will not be able to associate enjoyment with healthy nutrition. Most likely, every time this woman or man decides to "eat healthily," they will perform a ritual called "Say Goodbye to Delicious Food." This is the typical ritual of going all out, eating the favorite burger, desserts, and junk food, before starting the "good" diet on Monday. They will most likely overeat before even starting a diet plan and will most likely choose boring and tasteless food options in their new diet, increasing their chances of getting tired and quitting.

Which foods bring you pleasure at this moment?

_____

_____

_____

_____

What does eating healthy mean to you right now?

_____

_____

_____

_____

In this book, you will learn to enjoy healthy foods by choosing to do so mindfully. You will learn to choose healthy foods in accordance with your intentions.

Belief 2: The Most Delicious Food is Unhealthy Food

I have always loved chocolate. When I was younger, my father would sometimes take my sister and me to the corner store after lunch to buy us each a small piece of chocolate. It was shaped like a closed umbrella and wrapped in shiny, brightly colored foil.

I loved that chocolate umbrella!!!! But the store closed, and years passed. I grew up, moved to a different country where I tried dark Belgium chocolate. Oh my! Then a couple of years ago on a trip to Argentina, I found my beloved umbrella chocolates! Of course I bought them! The flavor was the same as I remember, but now it tasted awful. My taste buds tasted the low-quality ingredients of the chocolate. So, I threw away the horrible piece of "chocolate" and now treasure that memory with my father and sister for what it was: a family bonding moment.

Write a list of your favorite foods:

_____

_____

_____

_____

_____

I believe that if you try the same "foods," but have them made from better-quality ingredients, you will most likely change your preferences.

When you experiment with the quality of food you are eating, you will update your taste threshold. For example, if you feel like you cannot live without a McDonald's burger and fries, try to make your burger and fries at home with "real" ingredients. You will not only taste the difference, but you'll also *feel* the difference. Every step you make to choose healthier food will count. Start from where you are. Don't compare yourself to others, and don't rush.

For some people, it is time to find out how an organic apple tastes versus one grown from conventional agriculture. For others, it may be useful to experiment using water to satisfy their thirst rather than soda. Both steps are fantastic and essential. The point here is to get going. Experiment with your food by trying different textures and flavors. Upgrade the quality of your food. By doing this, you will reduce the amount of junk food you consume.

Another reason to upgrade the quality of your food is that it will help your body lower its toxic load. When your body is free from toxins, your taste buds will be cleaner and more efficient to taste. You will no longer need that vast amount of sugar in a cupcake to satisfy your need for something sweet. You will learn more on this topic in **Chapter 9, Tune-Up—Time to Detox.**

Your food choices change with time and depend on the percentage of quality food you choose to put in your body.

Ask yourself if there is a food that you didn't like as a child, but that you now love? List them here.

_____

_____

_____

When I was a child, I disliked eating vegetables because of their crunchy texture and the way they sounded when I chewed them. Now my diet is approximately 70-80 percent vegetables. To make this change, I had to explore ways to eat my veggies. First, I prepared them in soups or with creamy textures like mashes or as sauces. This way, I could start appreciating their taste and texture in a form I liked. Later, I experimented with other cooking methods and textures until I felt that I could eat some vegetables raw.

We tend to eat the same foods over and over just because it is all we know. I encourage you to experiment with food. Be brave! Try different recipes and cooking methods. For example, you may not like the smell of fish, but after eating a sushi roll, you may have a pleasant experience eating raw fish. That is a start! You may decide to experience fabulous

Peruvian "Nikkei Cuisine" or try a "Tiradito" or a "Ceviche." You may even learn that you like salmon or tuna just seared and sealed on the outside but raw on the inside. Be creative and allow yourself to play with tastes and textures!

Belief 3: Pleasure is a Bad Thing

Generations of people have been educated with guilt as their foundation. Therefore, the very concept of "pleasure" in many cultures is seen as wrong or even sinful. The predominantly Catholic belief that "pleasure is bad" still holds strong in the countries of South America. Every few months in North America, pop culture trendsetters label certain foods as "bad" and to "avoid at all costs." It is also undeniable that the entire world markets some foods as sinful temptations, or as being decadent.

This subliminal programming leads to the idea of good or bad foods, possibly making the act of eating something stressful for some (if not many) people. Guilt (when eating) could lead to a mindset that does not build a healthy relationship with food: "I will hide when I eat, so nobody knows how bad I am. I shouldn't eat that, and now I will punish myself." Punishment may be in the form of not eating, doing long and intense hours of exercise, vomiting or trying that new fad diet for the tenth time.

When you are eating, track your thoughts about food. What do you think about your meal? Does eating a particular food make you feel guilty? Do you think you deserve to eat enjoyable food? The key here is mindfulness and setting a strong intention. We will discuss this in **Chapter 5, Time for an Alignment—The Path of Mindfulness.**

Body-shaming doesn't help either. Our culture admires the under-weight model or TV star, the perfectly toned and photo-edited actor. These images have become the beauty standard. This standard makes a terrible contribution to society. Many people try to fit this standard, even if they have to be unhealthy to do it. Many people feel that anything is worth it if they could just have the body that would be visually qualified to be in a magazine.

Let me tell you something I learned before I took my personal food journey. Years ago, I worked in the TV and publicity industry. The goal of this industry is to sell, period, not to educate. They do not take responsibility for their influence. They are continually building this desirable world of "perfect-skinny-toned-happy-beautiful-successful" people to sell you something. From those role models, you will not get happiness nor healthy living.

We will talk more about this topic in **Chapter 13, Is My Vehicle Good Enough? Self-Image.** Meanwhile, ask yourself which desire is leading you when you make your food choices? Are you choosing to fit into an unreal beauty standard, or is it your desire to be healthy? What are your feelings about your choice? Anxiety, frustration, loneliness? It is OK to have these feelings, and it is essential to recognize them. This is the first step in your journey. A fascinating time!

To gain a healthier relationship with our food, we have to *incorporate* the idea that food *is* a pleasure. We experience the world through our senses, and we all begin life comforted by food. It is not about good or bad food; it is about choosing healthier, better quality, and yes—pleasurable—food that fuels your wellness. It is also about building a good relationship with food, one that nurtures you, empowers you, and elevates you.

Following is an exercise that will help you explore your relationship with food.

First: No judgment commitment

The first thing to do is to silence your inner judge. Instead of criticizing yourself, focus your thoughts toward curiosity and kindness. If you eat something you have previously considered "bad" or "unhealthy," all is not lost. Replace, "I broke my diet at the café with my friend. I should just give up," with "I had a nice time with my friend today, and this evening, I'll pass on dessert."

Be mindful of judging and imposing absolute rules on your food. Instead of saying, "I won't eat any more bread," try thinking, "I'll have some bread, but not so much as yesterday." For example, if someone wants to reduce their sugar consumption, they may feel they have to cut out all fruits and fruit juices right away. This type of "all or nothing" thinking tends to create decision-paralysis. Be gentle with yourself as you look at your food options.

Remember, every bite of food will become you. Your food becomes your blood, and then your cells. Therefore, investing in your relationship with food will result in having a better relationship with yourself.

Second: Food Journal

Track your eating habits, your food choices, and how you feel physically and emotionally after each meal or snack. Take a picture of each plate of food you eat so you can recall the portions. You will also want to write what you eat in a journal or in the **Your Personal Journey with Food, Food Journal**, which we have prepared for you at **www.journeywith-food.com**. At the end of the week, write your overall diet in your weekly **Your Personal Journal with Food Journal**. You will find this at the end of each chapter.

It is also essential to keep track of the environment in which you eat and the way you are eating. Who do you invite to your table: your cell phone, your TV, or a friend, family, or colleague? All this data will help you to see the way you are relating to your food.

Third: Every Week Explore Your Behavior Around Food

Every week go back through your journal. What do you see? Do you overeat? Do you even know if you are overeating? Do you hide when you eat? What healthy food makes you feel awesome? What unhealthy foods do you crave? What food makes you feel terrible?

Go deeper and explore your thoughts and emotions. Are there any thoughts or feelings that are leading you to eat? Do you feel guilty? The purpose of this exercise is to help you recognize behaviors that are contributing to an unhealthy relationship with food. By exposing these behaviors, you will be able to stop, cut that flow of energy, and replace those actions with new, healthy behaviors.

And remember, embrace that which is you! Embrace your journey!

Tracy and I will be with you every step of the way.

Your Personal Journal With Food

Week Number:_____ Date:_____

What did you eat this week?

_____

_____

_____

_____

_____

How many glasses of plain water per day?_____
Describe the environment in which you ate.

_____

_____

_____

_____

How were your behaviors around food?

_____

_____

What did you do this week that makes you happy?

_____

_____

What new foods, recipes, and cooking methods will you try next
week?

_____

_____

CHAPTER 2

Stuck on the Yo-Yo Diet Roundabout
By Tracy

Yo-Yos are toys. They were never intended to be defined as a troublesome path of diets and weight management. How many "diets" have you tried? One? Ten? Twenty-Five? For me, I have yo-yo'd so many times since my first "diet" in high school that it's difficult to count.

I have been frustrated so many times because I could not keep my weight—or waistline—under control. Because of that frustration and disappointment, I decided in my late 30s to early 40s to give up on myself. Luckily, I had a small voice speaking to me, from within telling me, "No! Don't give up! You can figure this out! You just don't know how yet. You can learn."

Guess what? I did learn, and so can you!

Many of my clients tell me that they are terrible people because they keep failing. Do you feel the same way? I sure did. Let's make an agreement that from this moment on, we will give ourselves some pats on the back and much deserved respect. Respect that we never gave up. Respect that we kept trying. Respect that we were and are NOT willing to give up on ourselves. Now that's pretty impressive!

How would it feel to know that you can unlock your body's secret to successful weight management? How beautiful would it be to be free from "diet" pressure? We are all different, and no single lifestyle diet is right for everyone. The foods and lifestyles that work for Ingrid and I are not necessarily going to work for you. What you find works for you will not necessarily work for me. And that's OK! Let's figure out what is right for YOU!

First of all, what exactly is a diet? Here are a few sources to help define "diet" for us:

The Merriam-Webster Dictionary defines a diet as:

A: *food and drink regularly provided or consumed*

B: *habitual nourishment*

C: *the kind and amount of food prescribed for a person or animal for a particular reason*

D: *a regimen of eating and drinking sparingly to reduce one's weight <going on a diet>*

Wikipedia defines a diet as:

a: *the sum of the food consumed by an organism or group.*

Did you notice anything while reading those definitions? We are ALL on diets! Every single one of us, every single day, is on some form of "diet." We all seek habitual nourishment, and we all partake in food and drink regularly. So, no big deal.

So, how does someone on a "diet" define "diet?"

A: *A frustrating amount of time filled with cravings, deprivation, and food I don't like, utilized to lose weight that I know I won't keep off, and/or;*

B: *Something I am doing right now because my doctor said I had to, and I can't wait to be off of it as soon as possible so I can eat what I want again.*

Do A and B sound familiar? They sure do to me!

One of the main reasons so many people struggle with their weight is that most people go on diets that do not work for their body or lifestyle. Everyone is very different and has different needs.

When we go on fad diets or crash diets to lose "weight," we damage our body. We can impair the body's ability to burn calories properly. Any education we receive during these diets does not carry over into real life and help us keep the weight off once we start bringing what we call "real" meals back into our daily routine.

I faced many challenges during my various "diets." These challenges came in different forms; cravings, hunger, anxiety, not knowing how to cook, missing my old ways, new habits, missing foods I had an emotional connection to, not losing weight fast enough, and being critical of myself. When I was on one of these fad diets, I harmed my body and morale more than helped them.

So how do you turn that Yo-Yo back into a child's toy? To do this, you need to do some homework and become a student of yourself. It's time to enjoy learning about your strengths as well as your shortcomings/weaknesses. You want to employ a journal for this. (If you haven't downloaded your complimentary **Your Personal Journal with Food** or **Your Personal Journey with Food Journal** yet, go to **www.journeywithfood.com** now to get your free pdf documents.

> "If you focus on results, you will never change.
> If you focus on change, you will get results."
>
> JACK DIXON

Steps to Letting Go of the Yo-Yo

Understand Body Composition vs. Weight: Most of us have a scale in our home. This scale can be a friend or a dark nightmare. I have had relationship issues with the scale most of my life, getting on it in the morning only to find that I am up yet another pound then feeling defeated and angry. Getting on it a week later, only to find I am still up more weight. I would get distraught with the scale. A standard scale is NOT my friend. The only scale I am willing to step on now is one that tells me my body composition and weight.

Remember that weight is one of many biomarkers associated with your health. Your body composition creates your weight. Your composition is everything that makes you, such as muscles, bones, brain matter, fat, cells, etc.

Two people can be the same height and weight, yet have entirely different body compositions. My recommendation: don't put your efforts just into losing weight on the scale, work on changing your body composition as well. When you do this, you have a higher chance of success. You will also be more apt to keep your healthy weight once attained.

Here is a list of just a few things that can modify your weight. The list is only a small glimpse, but I hope that it will start the dialogue within yourself to understand the many reasons your weight can change. (Sometimes overnight!)

- ⊕ Water Retention
- ⊕ Fat %
- ⊕ Muscle mass
- ⊕ Constipation
- ⊕ Dehydration
- ⊕ Bone density and size
- ⊕ Side effects of a food sensitivity or prescription drug

Chronic Restrictive Dieting: If you find that you are restricting yourself, take note of these symptoms. Chronic, restrictive dieting can cause the following symptoms, all of which can contribute to ill health.

- ⊕ Lowered Resting Metabolic Rate (5-10%, up to 15%)
- ⊕ Thyroid production impaired

- Sex hormone production impaired

- Constipation as the digestive system slows its pace to account for less food and the need to try and absorb as much nutrition as possible.

- Other symptoms associated with low micro-nutrients, such as being tired and "tingling" in hands and feet due to eating processed diet foods versus real, whole foods.

Understand the Path You Have Been On: Allow yourself to acknowledge the different diet programs you have tried. Note the challenges you have had. Note also what happened when these diet programs were "over." It is essential to write down everything you can, as these are clues that you can use to create a successful path moving forward. You must figure out what hasn't worked and what you thought did work in the past and why.

To help you brainstorm, I have jotted down a few of my experiences. These are just quick thoughts. You don't have to write in complete sentences. Just get the information down on paper, as I did below. Even toss in some of your thoughts about the situation as I have.

- My first diet at age 18, (1985/86), tried a liquid diet and protein shake diet, tasted awful and was hungry all the time. Quit.

- Baked potatoes were the health craze of the mid-'80s, ate a lot of them, didn't work, put on about 10-15 lbs.

- Non-fat diet, purchased only non-fat foods, etc.; didn't lose weight, gained weight, felt hungry all the time.

- PayDay candy bar and yogurt diet, age 19/20, anxiety-ridden, hungry, but looked good on the outside!

- Vegetarian diet (mostly processed vegetarian food) while exercising to the extreme, taking diet pills, looked FABULOUS, but was anxiety-ridden, heart rate issues caused by the diet pills. Still saw myself as not good enough. (Damn that cellulite on the outer part of my thighs! Why won't it go away!)

⊕ Restrictive caloric diet utilizing processed foods, hungry all the time, anxious and edgy, cravings, quit, and quickly gained about 5 lbs more above where I started.

⊕ 1990's USDA recommended dietary pyramid—gained about 10-15lbs! Felt like a failure, exercised every day like crazy, stressed to maintain. Once I stopped working out, I gained all the weight back and more. (Nutrition science is now proving that this dietary pyramid was flawed and has caused so many health problems for people.)

⊕ CR500 diet (Calorie Restricted, only 500 calories allowed each day) lost the weight, but had a hard time following the plan and strayed from it. Learned some great techniques on how to cook low-calorie meals. I gained all the weight back.

⊕ Wine/cheese/chocolate pairing diet—hmmm, gained about 20lbs with this one. Probably wasn't the best choice.

⊕ Meal Replacement Shakes; tried several over the past seven years. (I now know that whey protein is not an option for me as I have a high sensitivity to dairy. Whey gives me diarrhea and intestinal cramps. Now I use vegetarian protein powders mixed with fresh produce; mainly greens with a variety of other colorful vegetables and fruits. This is an excellent option for me.)

⊕ Lower carbohydrate, minimally refined foods, minimal to no added sugar, high veggie content, lean proteins. This is currently working for me! I am not on a strict paleo or ketogenic diet but have finally found the correct programming for my body to help me maintain a healthy weight. I still have ebbs and tides with my weight, but I am able to figure out what is happening with my body now. I can catch my behavior much sooner, isolate a food that may not be serving me, isolate a food that my body LOVES, figure out changes in my activity that may cause me to want more or less food. I am now aware. I am present. I am conscious with my body.

Please take some time right now to write down the experiences you've had with different diets by completing this next exercise.

Your History with Food Timeline

In the first column, list your various ages, from infant to now. If you are 40 years old, you will have 0-40 listed numerically, or you can break it down into fewer year spans, such as 2-5 years.

Next to your age ranges, in the second column, write down how you were fed as a child and how you fed yourself. Note what your favorite foods were and any weight changes you recall.

Now in the third column, write the significant emotional things that you have been through during those time frames: relationships with parents, siblings, school issues, marriage, divorce, moving, children, employment, even hormonal changes in puberty, pregnancy, menopause as appropriate to your case.

In the fourth column, write what type of exercise, sports, and level of physical activity you may have participated in at those times.

This exercise will allow you to see why you are where you are. You may see some relationship between healthy habits, foods, and emotions. You may notice that during times when you were very active, you were eating a certain way, but when things changed, and your activity dropped, you kept the same foods in your life and may have gained weight. This is your food history, and you will utilize it for learning. Using it, along with this book, will improve your health.

History With Food Timeline

AGE	DIETS/FOODS	LIFE MILESTONES	EXERCISE

AGE	DIETS/FOODS	LIFE MILESTONES	EXERCISE

My main struggle with dieting and why it has never worked long-term for me was that I didn't understand the various reasons I gained the weight. And when I did lose weight, I didn't really understand why. **Let me repeat that: I didn't understand the various reasons I gained the weight. And when I did lose weight, I didn't really understand why.** It wasn't clear to me how food affected me, not only on the bathroom scale but also in how I felt physically and emotionally. I also didn't understand why I was making certain food choices. I hadn't learned how to live a healthy lifestyle. I didn't even know what a healthy lifestyle was, let alone what one would look like for ME. I used food to comfort me in times of stress and anxiety. I would also stop eating during times of stress and anxiety. It all depended on the situation. I continued to fall back into old habits that were so much "easier," even though they were much "harder" on my body and mind.

It is vital to study yourself regarding past dieting and weight gain/loss. Acknowledge where you have been, what has and hasn't worked, and what ultimately derailed you from your plan. By doing this, you can figure out the "why" and, therefore, your next steps. Weight loss success is much more than just how many calories you burn and consume. Hormones, genetics, genetic expression, your environment, gut health and nutrient absorption, the type of calories, physical stress, and emotional stress all play a part. We have to acknowledge this.

To help you begin figuring out what your next steps will be, review the following questions. Give yourself the opportunity to answer them. Give yourself the opportunity to answer each question to its fullest.

What healthy lifestyle habits and behaviors do I currently have, and when and why did I implement them?

_____

_____

_____

_____

_____

What not-so-healthy lifestyle habits and behaviors do I currently have, and when and why did I implement them?

_____

_____

_____

_____

_____

What food choices am I making? Do I understand the impact these foods have on my body, positively or negatively? Do I know what foods support me best? Do I know which ones do not support me?

_____

_____

_____

_____

_____

Could I have an underlying health issue to address, such as pre-diabetes, type 2 diabetes, heart disease, thyroid dysfunction, adrenal fatigue, irritable bowel syndrome, heart disease, or something else?

_____

_____

_____

_____

_____

When was the last time I went to see a doctor?

_____

_____

_____

_____

_____

Am I afraid of going to the doctor because I'm afraid of what they may find and knowing it could mean having to change?

_____

_____

_____

_____

Do I know what the following information means? Hemoglobin A1C(HBA1c); fasting glucose; fasting insulin; vitamins; minerals; and hormone levels?

_____

_____

_____

_____

Why do I eat?

_____

_____

_____

_____

What drives my food choices?

_____

_____

_____

_____

_____

Do I know enough about the food I am choosing to eat?

_____

_____

_____

_____

Am I not eating enough?

_____

_____

_____

_____

Could I be undernourished even though I am getting plenty of calories?
Do I know what this question means?

_____

_____

_____

_____

Am I giving my body the opportunity for movement?

_____

_____

_____

_____

Am I covering up an emotional pain that I have yet to address?

_____

_____

_____

_____

Am I on a prescription that has side effects such as reduced nutrient absorption, weight gain, or water retention? If so, is it possible to modify my doses by working with my doctor? Can I get a plan put together with my doctor so that I can stop taking this prescription? Have I asked my doctor about alternatives?

_____

_____

_____

_____

Do I believe that being hungry is an emergency? If yes, why? If no, why?

_____

_____

_____

_____

Now that you have answered these questions, how do you feel? I hope that you are beginning to get a clear picture of what is happening for you. You have started your first step at being mindful. You will be learning about mindfulness in this book. Mindfulness is the beginning of a new life for you. Mindfulness has changed me forever, and I am most grateful for having been taught this skill.

We are a society of people intent on pursuing "instant gratification" in many ways, and "going with the flow." We don't pay attention. We can miss the fact that the weight we've gained probably happened over some years and all the situations that life brings that may have caused us to lose our way. It can be a challenge to acknowledge that the true journey you must now take is to reverse years of accumulated stress and weight that has brought your body to its current state.

Here are areas in your life where you will begin to apply the tools of mindfulness, thus allowing you to stop yoyo dieting.

Honor Your Body

I finally came to terms with the fact that my body is ALWAYS doing the best it can with what I am providing it and doing to it. I am not in denial anymore, and I no longer get angry with my body or myself. I finally honor my body and give it the respect it deserves for keeping me alive as best it can. A big realization that has helped me is to know that my body doesn't know how to handle most processed foods. When I eat now, I ask myself if the food I am choosing honors what my body can do or not. I also thank it for carrying me through my days and nights. I am mindful of the fact that my body inhales oxygen and then exhales. What miracles does your body perform for you on a daily basis? See if you can come up with a minimum of ten. Go ahead and jot these down here or in your journal. Please don't skip the exercise. Your mind will better acknowledge all the positive things your body does for you when you write them down.

_____

_____

_____

_____

_____

Isn't it amazing what your body does for you? Let's give it some love and respect! Take a moment and say this to your body, I know you may feel silly, but say it with a smile on your face and with love in your heart.

"Body, you are amazing! Thank you for all you do for me every single day of my life! I love you and appreciate you so much! I commit to taking excellent care of you as you are a priceless miracle!"

"Ahhhhhh! You are welcome!" Your body sighs and loves your right back!

(Consider saying this to your body every single day. What amazing things can happen for your body when you say this to it every day? I believe that many amazing, wonderful things will happen for it AND for you!)

Skills

We will go into further details in future chapters, but here is a list of skills you will be learning and utilizing on *Your Personal Journey with Food*.

Listen: Your body sends you signals every single day, every moment. Listening and then responding appropriately to these messages will open a whole new world for you. Listening to your body is key to maintaining a healthy weight and lifestyle. Look for clues: Are you stressed? How does the food you eat make you feel during and after your meal? Do you have aches and pains that prevent you from exercising? Can you get help with these or find another way to begin moving? Take a moment to scan over your body from head to toe mentally. Write down what you notice. Get detailed. How does your scalp feel? Your jaw? Your ears? Go step by step, bone by bone, joint by joint, internal organs, scan everything from head to toe. What do you notice? Write it down here.

_____

_____

_____

_____

_____

Be Willing to Grow as a Person: Be willing to grow into whom you need to be to make life-lasting changes. Be willing to step into the new you and embrace this person with open arms. Thank the person you are. Thank the person you have been. Thank the person you have been for doing the best you could with what you knew. Thank your body for doing the best it could under the circumstances. Thank your "self" for stepping into your new life. Thank your "self" for buying this book! Do you have a vision of who you want to become? Take a moment to write down this vision of your future self. Once done, invite this person to join you on this journey right now. Let this person help guide you. Let this person help make decisions that support you.

_____

_____

_____

_____

_____

Sleep: I prided myself on my supposed ability to function on 5 hours or less of sleep per night. I was a "super-human" because I didn't need to sleep. Sleep was for the weak. Well, I was wrong. Sleep is one of the most essential parts of a healthy lifestyle and supportive diet regimen. What's happening regarding your sleep patterns right now? Do you need to make changes to your schedule to allow for more sleep? Do you have insomnia or sleep apnea? What can you do to help yourself settle into a good night's rest? We will discuss more in **Chapter 12, Rest Stop—Time to Get Some Much-Needed Sleep.**

_____

_____

_____

_____

_____

Stress: Do you have a great deal happening in your life right now, which makes you feel anxiety or distress? Do these circumstances cause you to eat, or do you not eat? Be sure to analyze this. Note below on a scale of 1-10 your stress levels and what is causing them at this time. Also, note if you tend to eat or not when you are distressed. We will discuss more in **Chapter 11—Emergency! I'm Stuck at Full Throttle!—Stress.**

_____

_____

_____

_____

_____

Cravings: Look at them as valuable information. What foods do you crave, and when do you crave them? Cravings can lead you to your solutions! Take a moment to jot down any cravings you have. We will discuss more in **Chapter 6, Your Journey Buddies—Symptoms as a Co-Pilot.**

_____

_____

_____

_____

Label Reading: As will be discussed in **Chapter 10, An Important Detour—The Controversies of Food** become a label reading guru! Investigate all that you put into your priceless body. How confident are you at reading labels, and how often do you read them before purchasing a product?

_____

_____

_____

_____

_____

How to Get Started

Pick from the list below and begin adding these healthy lifestyle changes into your life. I recommend starting with drinking plenty of water. (You will be surprised how well your body responds when it receives enough water!) Then choose the next lifestyle change and add that into your new routine. Get settled with one item before moving on and adding the next. The time it takes to implement lifestyle changes is different for everyone. Be patient! Don't give up on yourself. You are not in a race! Look at your calendar and create a plan as to when you want to add one of these new skills.

Drink Plenty of Water: Your body is approximately 60% water. The body cannot function without water. Dehydration makes it challenging to lose weight because you need it to help flush out waste that is produced by burning calories and fat. Water also helps curb appetite.

Eat the Rainbow: A plate of veggies and fruits gives the body the nutrients it needs to function. If you are eating minimal calories in an attempt to shed some pounds, but they are minimal calories from processed foods, your body is going to be starving nutritionally. By eating a rainbow of veggies and fruits, your body will begin to feel satisfied, and your cravings will diminish.

Eat Protein: There is much debate out on the internet as to what is the best protein to consume. Again, everyone is different, and bodies react differently to different foods. Use mindfulness to figure out your body. We recommend high-quality lean proteins and vegetable proteins. Go to **www.journeywithfood.com**, and you will find a link to a free pdf you can download showing protein options.

Become Your Own Chef: Learn to cook. Store simple, real food staple items so that you can have them on hand and ready to go at a moment's notice. I like to batch cook, then freeze or can, my meals for later. (Cook once, eat three or more times.) By batch cooking, I not only save time, but I also save money.

Crowd-Out: Make more time for supportive habits and less time for those that cause harm to you mentally and physically. In regard to your food, eat more whole foods, less refined and processed foods. Watch less TV, take more walks outside, for example.

Balance Blood Sugar: Integrate whole food snacks into your daily routine if you find that you are overly hungry between meals. You can download a handout with some excellent ideas at **www.journeywithfood.com**.

Build Physical Strength and Stamina: Allow time for physical activity. Create movement in your life and create a mind-body connection within that movement.

Address Silent Inflammation: Remove inflammatory foods from your diet, such as sugar, refined carbohydrates, and processed foods. Increase your intake of Omega-3 fatty acids, add in healthy fats, and remove trans-fats. Go to **www.journeywithfood.com** and download a free PDF for more information.

Get Blood Work Panels Done: Get your nutrient, hormone, and blood sugar levels checked. See Dr. Hyman's book referenced below. There is a wealth of information in this book on what blood work you should have done and why. Although this book focusses on Type 2 Diabetes, much of it will also pertain to your overall health. After all, the body is many "systems" working together. Type 2 Diabetes is a symptom of the system not functioning at its' optimal level.

HOW TO WORK WITH YOUR DOCTOR AND GET WHAT YOU NEED, by Dr. Hyman. You can download it for free at https://drhyman.com/wp-content/uploads/2012/04/HowToGet-WhatYouNeed.pdf.

Hire an Integrative Nutrition Health Coach: Entering into a new lifestyle can be an overwhelming experience. With guidance, you can learn to settle into your new lifestyle with confidence and less stress. Feel free to reach out to us at **start@journeywithfood.com.**

Your Personal Journal With Food

Week Number:_____ Date:_____

What did you eat this week?

_____

_____

_____

_____

_____

How many glasses of plain water per day? _____
What did you do this week that makes you happy?

_____

_____

_____

Describe the environment in which you ate.

_____

_____

How were your behaviors around food?

_____

_____

From the list below, which did you choose to do last week?

Drink plenty of water		Balance Blood Sugar	
Eat the Rainbow		Build Strength and Stamina	
Become your own chef		Address Silent Inflammation	
Crowd-Out		Eat Lean Protein	

How did it go? Did anything get in the way? What challenges came up?

_____

_____

_____

Which of the following are you going to experiment with next week?

Drink plenty of water		Balance Blood Sugar	
Eat the Rainbow		Build Strength and Stamina	
Become your own chef		Address Silent Inflammation	
Crowd-Out		Eat Lean Protein	

What challenges may occur in your life and schedule that could make it difficult to be successful? Utilize your experience from last week and see if there is a way you can modify your plan to allow yourself time for success. Do you need to block out time on your calendar? Do you need to go to the grocery store at a different time? Do you need assistance from others? Write down any situations that could make it difficult for you to move forward with your plan and do your best to be solution-oriented so that you can be successful.

_____

_____

_____

_____

_____

How did it go?

_____

_____

_____

Which of the following are you going to experiment with in the next two weeks?

Drink plenty of water		Balance Blood Sugar	
Eat the Rainbow		Build Strength and Stamina	
Become your own chef		Address Silent Inflammation	
Crowd-Out		Eat Lean Protein	

How did it go?

CHAPTER 3

_____

_____

_____

On the Road with Your Map and GPS
By Ingrid

GPS is an excellent tool to use when you want to get to a specific destination. You can see your route and even have information available about traffic that can lead to better choices on when to leave home and which direction to take.

When you are on a journey with food, it is essential to have something like a GPS to guide you every step of the way. The reason most diets fail is that there is no roadmap, no GPS. The problem is not your lack of motivation. You need a customizable system that goes with you through your journey. A tool to measure where you are, indicate your destination, and help you navigate along the way. In this chapter, you will explore some tools that will help you find your inner GPS.

First, you need to set your location. Is it possible to get somewhere if you don't know where you are? We have to know where we are to begin a journey. On this food journey, we will find our starting point by being very honest about what we are eating.

If you are what you eat, then who are you? You literally are what you have eaten and absorbed.

- ⊕ You are soda
- ⊕ You are candy
- ⊕ You are veggies
- ⊕ You are fruits
- ⊕ You are junk food
- ⊕ You are whole foods

The well-known saying, "You are what you eat," is used frequently to promote a healthy lifestyle, but what does the saying mean? It means that all the nutrients, minerals, and vitamins from your food will become your blood, which then becomes your cells, which becomes you. This is why food quality matters so much.

Modern science backs up this idea. "The brain is the result of what we eat," according to the Chilean investigator Fernando Gómez Pinilla, a UCLA professor of neurosurgery and physiological science and a member of UCLA's Brain Research Institute and Brain Injury Research Center.

"Food is like a pharmaceutical compound that affects the brain," says Gómez-Pinilla. "Diet, exercise, and sleep have the potential to alter our brain health and mental function. This all raises the exciting possibility that changes in diet are a viable strategy for enhancing cognitive abilities, protecting the brain from damage and counteracting the effects of aging."[1]

For example, Omega 3 fatty acids, and especially DHA, are like building blocks for the brain. Their benefits are many, such as improved learning and memory and their ability to fight against mental disorders such as depression and mood disorders, schizophrenia, and dementia.

---

1. The original link to this interview is no longer working and was on the UCLA web page. You may find a similar interview at https://www.livescience.com/2675-good-diet-exercise-brain-healthy.html The analysis of the 160 studies about food's effect on the brain is published in the 2008 July issue of the journal Nature Reviews Neuroscience.

In contrast to the health effects of diets that are rich in omega-3 fatty acids, studies indicate that diets high in trans fats and saturated fats (found in many processed foods) adversely affect cognition. In other words, your ability to reason, learn, and remember is literally affected by the food you eat!

How does low-quality food affect your brain? According to Daniel Amen, MD, junk food and fast food negatively affect brain synapses and specific molecules related to learning and memory. Excessive caloric intake, most common in junk food, can reduce the flexibility of synapses and increase the vulnerability of cells to damage by causing the formation of free radicals.

Free radicals are single atoms with unpaired electrons. Electrons like to be in pairs, so these atoms "steal" that missing electron from a neighbor cell so they can become a pair. This process creates more free radicals and large chain chemical reactions in your body. These reactions are called oxidation and cause damage to cells, fatty tissue, proteins, and DNA. Oxidation damage is associated with chronic diseases like type 2 diabetes, high blood pressure, heart disease, cancer, and others. They also may have a link to aging. Moderate caloric intake could protect the brain by reducing oxidative damage to cellular proteins, lipids, and nucleic acids.

This is all to say that your body and mind will respond to any change in your eating patterns. Don't worry if you've eaten fast food on a regular basis. You always have the power, time, and ability to improve your health and brain cells.

Have you heard about the theory that every seven years your body builds new cells? To prove this, Dr. Jonas Frisen and a team of Swedish researchers from the Karolinska Institute in Stockholm, measure the age of cells in the body using the same method used in archaeology and paleontology to pinpoint the age of fossils. They discovered that cells renew themselves over various periods of time, depending on their kind. Look at their fascinating findings:

A) Epidermis cells (which make up the skin of our bodies and is our barrier to the environment) are recycled every couple weeks;

B) Red blood cells last four months, and then renew;

C) The body's detoxifier is the liver and liver cells last between 300 to 500 days;

D) Cells within the surface of the intestinal lining are among the shortest-lived in the entire body, surviving for only five days. However, the average age of other intestinal cells is 15.9 years;

E) Skeletal system cells last just over ten years while cells of the rib muscles average 15.1 years;

F) The brain cells of the visual cortex, the area responsible for sight, were as old as the test subject themselves. These cells do not regenerate. Other brain cells have a shorter lifespan;

G) The heart as a whole does generate new cells, but the investigators could not yet measure the turnover rate;

H) The average age of an adult's body cellular system may be as young as 7 to 10 years.

The body is continually renewing itself, disposing of, and building new cells daily. Therefore, the quality of nutrients in our diets is critical. These nutrients are the building blocks for cell growth and repair. Thus, we have the opportunity to improve our health and energy every time we eat. This is great news! The decision is always yours. Every time you choose something to eat, you are building the future you.

Exercise: Awareness—Calibrate Your GPS

Now is an excellent time to see what you are in relation to what you eat! Before continuing with this chapter, we invite you to take this book with you, go to your pantry and refrigerator, explore everything there, and answer the following questions:

What are the products you eat most frequently?

What is accumulating dust?

What is the percentage of packaged food versus whole foods?

How much produce, dairy, meat, and processed foods are you consuming?

How many products do you have with strange ingredients?

How many sugary or hidden sugar products do you see?

Do you eat mostly fresh food or frozen, boxed, and reheated food?

Remember knowing where you are will:
1. Tell you what you need to address so that you can start your journey; and
2. Help you as a reference point to see your improvements and motivate you to keep going.

As you advance through this program, pay attention to your body's signals. Sometimes we make decisions on what we think our body needs, but what we choose could be the opposite of what it needs.

Set Your Destination

So, if you are what you eat, what do you want to be? As you know by now, healthier food choices can help you to get closer to becoming the person you want to be. Defining that destination is essential. What do you want to experience in your life by having a healthier relationship with food? How will you feel if food empowers you?

We recommend you visualize your destination instead of setting a goal. Why visualize a destination instead of setting a goal? Visualizing a destination is to see yourself living your life, eating healthy, feeling comfortable in your body. It is to integrate every aspect of your life. When a person is asked to set a goal, that goal is of logical construction and comes from the left side of the brain.

In theory, every food plan or diet works, but what happens when you try to apply theory into your everyday life? The fail rate of "that plan" increases because, as a society, we use food to make bonds, to socialize, even to fall in love. Just think about birthday celebrations, anniversary dinners, chat and coffee, family brunches, Thanksgiving, and Christmas. We do not eat to survive; we add emotions to our food.

When an emotional component is involved, such as food choices or habits, the path becomes tricky. The route can be filled with U-turns, circles, and detours. It is not a straight line going from point A to point B. Your GPS might have you going in circles! With emotions, you may use food to make yourself feel better or to fill emotional needs, rather than to nurture your body. Not being aware of your feelings in terms of food could lead to emotional eating. Emotional eating is when your emotions, not your hunger, decide what, when, and how much you will eat. For example, you are in a restaurant and already satisfied with the main dish, but you "make room" for dessert because it looks fabulous and everybody at the table will have dessert. In this scenario, you are motivated by a need to fit in, not because you are hungry. How about when you are about to accomplish a challenging task and feel the need for something crunchy, or the times you feel sad and try to comfort yourself with ice cream or chocolate or alcohol. All these actions are taken because of a feeling, not a need to fuel your body. Physical food will never fill a void of emotional hunger.

There is a difference between the emotional link we all establish with food and emotional eating. In the first case, you will eat until you are satisfied, for example, think of a baby. When a baby breastfeeds, it will stop eating when full. This is quite different from compulsive behavior motivated by filling some emptiness, pain, or unresolved feeling—for example, a person who binge eats. Binge eating does not build any connection with other people; it is often done as a solitary act that involves shame and guilt. Binge eating involves a disconnect between your true feelings and your self-awareness.

Emotions can be measured by vibratory frequency. We have high-frequency emotions like confidence, love, joy, hope, peace, and low-frequency emotions: shame, fear, anger, envy, sadness. High-frequency emotions are just like dense-nutritious-packed food. There is no need to overeat because you are feeling incredible, and you will like to stay that way. Know that if you are feeling low, you don´t have to feed into those feelings. You can learn to elevate the frequency by using the exact thing you need: love, self-love to be precise. Your first true and long-lasting love is to yourself, so if you are not feeling well, the best way out is to take care of you: pick healthy food, sleep enough, move your body.

The key here is to recognize which feelings are driving your eating. Does food comfort and nurture you until you are satisfied, or do you feel the way you eat is not respecting your body. Remember that food creates relationships, not only with others but with you.

How do you get along with yourself?

_____

_____

_____

What kind of relationship are you building through eating?

_____

_____

_____

Is your food a healthy supply of fuel, allowing you to feel good so that you can do the things that make you happy, or do you eat so much that almost all your energy is utilized for digestion, and you feel sick?

_____

_____

_____

Any answer is correct. To know where you are is the first step. We will help you with that.

On the following page is an exercise that will allow you to EXPLORE YOUR RELATIONSHIP WITH FOOD.

Exercise: Build Your Road Map

1. Visualize your destination. What do you want to experience in your life by having a healthier relationship with food?

_____

_____

_____

_____

_____

2. Grab **Your Personal Journal with Food** and read your notes. Do you see any patterns? What have you discovered in the following areas?

The number of healthy foods you are eating: _____

The number of unhealthy foods you are eating: _____

The frequency of eating: _____

How are your habits? Can you identify a trigger that leads you to healthy or unhealthy food choices?

_____

_____

_____

_____

Can you pick a food habit to improve?

_____

_____

_____

_____

If you have done that, then you have found one of the first destinations on your journey.

The key to setting the coordinates on your personal GPS is consciousness. To find your current "location," you need to be aware of what you eat every day and recognize the feelings you experience every time you eat. Are you hungry? Are you bored? Are you anxious? Are you thirsty? Be aware of your needs: do you need a hug or a doughnut?

Recalculating…

You will achieve the best results when your strategy includes mistakes and "falling off the wagon" as a way to learn. Many times, my clients (and even I) feel the pressure of achieving an outcome. Therefore, we don't pay attention to the process that the path is teaching.

For example, somebody wants to lose 5 pounds immediately with a FAD diet. This person is successful at losing the 5 pounds, but after a few months, reverts to old habits and gains the weight back. During the diet, that person only focused on the results (losing 5 pounds) and getting there fast. They didn't learn how to maintain the lasting effects, nor did they learn how to build a healthier relationship with food. So, every time that person wants to lose weight, they are trapped in that spiral.

Remember that life will happen on your journey with food, and you will learn how to deal with unplanned changes in a proactive way. What if you focus on what you will gain instead of what you may be losing? You are gaining a new experience with food that leads to a healthy and sustainable lifestyle. Once you focus on gaining, the experience will be your teacher, and your chances of building long-lasting habits will increase.

Now that you have your destination set in your mind, start to record your action steps in your journal.

What can you do today to improve *Your Personal Journey with Food?*

_____

_____

_____

⊛ Maybe you will need to prepare your meals in advance and take them with you so you will reduce eating fast food.

⊛ Maybe you have to review a restaurant on the internet before choosing to dine and make sure it will cover your needs.

⊛ Maybe you have to learn some new recipes.

Instead of regretting or blaming an unplanned situation that caused you to break your plan, you will learn to be proactive and come up with new solutions. These new solutions will get you back on your path fast. This behavior will allow you to get closer to your destination. Those "new solutions" will be your action steps, your map. Be mindful and observe to make sure those steps are taking you where you want to go. And remember, you can modify your steps along the way if necessary. If one day you don't accomplish your action step, make a note and ask yourself why not, and what you can do better next time. This way, you will not waste any time feeling guilty. You will use your time in a smart and self-supportive way.

Go ahead. Focus on your actions and be consistent. By focusing on small steps and actions you take every day, you will ultimately arrive at your destination.

Remember: By honoring your food, you honor your body. By choosing wisely for your body and health, you will be honoring yourself.

Your Personal Journal With Food

Week Number:_____   Date:_____

What did you eat this week?

_____

_____

_____

_____

_____

How many glasses of plain water per day?_____
What did you do this week that makes you happy?

_____

_____

How are your habits? Can you identify a trigger that leads you to
healthy or unhealthy food choices?

_____

_____

Monday: What can I do today to improve my relationship with food?

_____

_____

Tuesday: What can I do today to improve my relationship with food?

_____

_____

Wednesday: What can I do today to improve my relationship with food?

_____

_____

Thursday: What can I do today to improve my relationship with food?

_____

_____

Friday: What can I do today to improve my relationship with food?

_____

_____

Saturday: What can I do today to improve my relationship with food?

_____

_____

Sunday: What can I do today to improve my relationship with food?

CHAPTER 4

_____

_____

Choosing the "Scenic Route" Instead of the "Fast Track"

By Ingrid

When you're driving along a beautiful route, everything in your vehicle needs to be working well, to concentrate better on the view! You don't want to be distracted by a strange noise in the engine, or a "low fuel" light, or an unpredictable backseat driver. All of these factors can be important to help us enjoy the scenery.

What do you have to do with your diet to better enjoy your health journey? Western cultures tend to look at only some components of food and nutrition, such as calories, proteins, carbohydrates, and fats to understand food. However, nutrition is much more than just the components in food. Nutrition is also about variety, combinations, digestion, chewing, your mood, and a lot more.

It may take some time for us to see our bodies and health as a whole concept because we are in the habit of seeing them in segmented ways. This is due in part to the way "nutrition" and "health" are conceptualized and also marketed. We have expert doctors who specialize in each organ or body system. We have products designed for specific people and different areas of the body. The vitamin aisle is a perfect example of this, displaying different vitamins for men, women, children, nails, skin, brain, bones, bowel, etc. There are thousands of articles and studies on "good-food-for-something-specific" that influence the discussion about food and market preferences. And, there are a lot of foods and products claiming to be the best. "The most potent antioxidant." "The protein with the best absorption." "The lowest-GI carbohydrate." These products remain at the top for a couple of months until a new product from a more exotic origin replaces them. The result is lots of confusion about nutrition, and increased consumption that benefits only the "health food" industry.

Your body is made up of many parts, but you are more than just your parts. Each part works with the others as a team; there is some intelligence that makes all the organs work without you having to worry about them. Your body takes all the actions required to keep you alive without you having to think about it. So much importance is given to the "parts" that we forget the fundamental concept of holistic health. Holistic health combines all the details and parts, making it possible to organize them into one picture.

"Holistic" health is synergistic. It combines all the physical parts with emotional and mental health, to visualize "synergy" in a person. What is synergy?

Synergy: The interaction of two or more agents or forces so that their combined effect is greater than the sum of their individual effects.

Your body "parts" work together in synergy. A perfect example that demonstrates this synergy is the connection between the brain, the bowels, and the immune system. The complete digestive system of the body runs from the esophagus to the anus. Forming a unique anatomic unity that is called the "enteric nervous system," and just like the brain, has nerve fibers running throughout it. This system controls the whole digestive process, including nutrient absorption and peristaltic movement (contractions of the esophagus and intestines that move food), and collaborates with the body's immune system. The same hormones and neurotransmitters are found in the brain and the gut, like dopamine and serotonin, among others. Those substances are related to our mood, happiness level, sleep patterns, and regulates hunger, body temperature, and other body functions.

Within our gut live microbiota, a whole microscopic world, whose population is ten times the amount of our body cells. These friendly bacteria help us to finish digestion, feed us, and protect us. They are the first line of defense against unfriendly bacteria.

Symptoms of illness are not usually due to just one thing. We function and experience life inside this system. One that is holistically created of many parts and synergistically operates as a whole. All parts are dependent on the other. Everything is integral to everything else. Synergy is the reason we should pay attention not only to our food calories but to the quality of those calories. We need to pay attention to the way we prepare our food, how, why, and when we eat it, how we chew it, and how we digest it.

The body is a fantastic system, and each organ has a specific and vital role that could be affected if another is not functioning well.

Scenic Overlook: Don't Just Feed the Body, Feed the Soul

We know that we are more than our bodies and that we experience life on many other levels, not just the physical. Emotions nurture us just like food does. Our emotions can be superfoods that elevate our spirit, or they can be like junk food that depletes our energy. Have you ever experienced indigestion after eating something because, earlier in the day, you had a rough discussion or argument with a loved one? Have you ever felt so full of energy and mental clarity by doing something that you felt much passion about, even after spending all day without eating anything? Emotions are a powerful source of energy that feeds our mental, spiritual, emotional, and physical being. Perhaps you can think of emotions as a passenger in your car on your lifelong journey of health. This passenger can easily make the journey more enjoyable, but at times our emotions will convert into a dreaded backseat driver!

When we look at our food and our lives from a holistic perspective, things that happen to us, which have no calories nor physical ingredients, become nutrition for the soul, the heart, the mind. These experiences comfort and ease our hunger and thirst for love. They propel us into doing fun things or going on an adventure. Instead of gorging yourself on food, gorge yourself on life, and satisfy every level of hunger!

Understanding holistic nutrition in this way helps us consider and understand how we are nurturing our whole life in general:

> Am I feeling supported?
>
> Do I have people in my life that I trust?
>
> What can I share in order to have satisfying relationships?
>
> What is a fulfilling career, and how can I like mine more?
>
> Do I live according to my spiritual beliefs?
>
> Am I happy and comfortable with my partner, family, work, and body? What do I have to do or change to achieve that?
>
> How can I spend my time so that I can have my dream life?
>
> What kind of emotional food does my soul need?

Recognize yourself as a WHOLE being. The way you experience your life (and how that way of being combines with food) gives you a powerful tool to take the wheel and drive you to where you want to go. Finding and creating the answers to these questions will help you make and sustain positive changes to your lifestyle.

Whole Foods

Hippocrates was right in saying that food is medicine, but food by itself isn't a magic pill!

Throughout this chapter, we've discussed how food and nutrition work in synergy with all the parts of your being. Nutrition is not about adding everything marketed to us as healthy to our diet. It's not specifically about "organic produce" or some trendy super-food. Due to so many products and conflicting information available, people get confused as to what they should eat. I even notice that some people get very distressed about their food because they may be doing something wrong like they will be punished!

Many of my clients come to me, asking if a particular food is healthy, or if they should eat more of a specific super-food or what to eat to overcome something specific. My reply is always to look at the whole picture. If you are currently getting 95 percent of your nutrition from junk foods such as fried foods, sandwiches, processed meats, and sugary stuff, then add a nutritious vegan protein shake, packed with super-foods and antioxidants to your diet, you are not going to improve your health in the long term. It is a positive step, of course! But to see changes, you need to dramatically increase the nutritious whole foods you are eating while reducing processed foods from your diet.

The Source of Your Food Matters

If the core of your diet consists of sugar bombs made from organic sugarcane, dates, nut butter, blueberries, cacao nibs, maca powder, spirulina, and other healthy ingredients, you are still building a diet from snacks and bread! This will not improve your health!

When you eat a diet that is 75-90 percent whole foods such as fresh produce and no processed foods, the healthy ingredients will work better because you will be creating a synergy. If you are not eating 75-90 percent of whole foods in your weekly diet, there's no need to panic. The most permanent change is a slow, gradual change.

Exercise: Photo Opportunity on the Scenic Route

Let's take a quick stop to see where you are! Review the list of foods you ate last week in **Your Personal Journal with Food** and calculate the percentage of processed foods. Remember, processed foods are those that have gone through a mechanical or chemical process to change or preserve it. Typically, they come in a box or bag and have more than one item on the ingredients list.

This week, my percentage of processed food is:_____%

What Is "Healthy?" What Are Whole Foods?

There's an easy answer to that question: as long as the food looks more like it does in nature, it is a whole food and better for your body. And preparing homemade food from whole foods will always be better than pre-packaged, processed food.

For example, take wheat. With all the gluten-free products these days, it seems like wheat is the latest villain of our times. But is it the wheat? The food industry has made massive varieties of products that contain wheat and flour, which has increased the amount of wheat and gluten we eat. You may find gluten not only in cereal and bread. You will find it in foods that shouldn't have it at all, like dairy and sugar products. What matters is the overall amount of it that you eat.

Eating cooked wheat grain (called mote in Chile and wheat berry in the USA) adds fiber and magnesium to your diet, but eating white flour elevates your glucose levels in the blood and, therefore usually, insulin levels. As I said before, it is a matter of quality and source or origin.

Eating food that is, and looks, closer to nature is going to be more nutritious. After all, maybe there is a strong reason why we cannot find powdered wheat (flour) in nature?

So, how about creating a virtuous circle in your life by improving your food quality? Choosing whole foods is a matter of self-care and practicing self-love. Nutrition works in synergy, just like you do, and it will make a positive impact on the whole you.

List of Whole Foods

Proteins

Animal proteins: grass-fed beef, free-range and grain-fed chicken, fish (be sure to take a moment to review the Environmental Working Group's list of low mercury fish on their web page), pork, seafood, lamb, rabbit, turkey, etc.

Plant-based proteins: legumes (lentils, garbanzo, beans, peanut, peas), quinoa, kale, fermented soy products.

Carbohydrates
Whole grains (corn, millet, oats, buckwheat, wheat, brown rice, and other grains not flour!), potatoes, sweet potatoes, yucca, or mandioca.

Vegetables
All kinds of green leaves, herbs, celery, cucumber, broccoli, cauliflower, zucchini, eggplant, cabbage, pumpkin, carrots, onion, garlic, mushrooms, etc.

Fruits
All kinds, including tomatoes and avocados.

Fats
Seeds, avocados, nuts, olives, olive oil, coconut oil, and avocado oil.

Exercise: Adding Whole Foods

1. Pick two foods from each category from the previous list of whole foods and add those to any meal this week. Write your choices here.

_____

_____

_____

_____

_____

2. See your list of favorites foods in **Chapter 1, Before You Start Your Journey**. Are there whole foods on that list? Can you find a recipe in which you can create the same flavor, but in a healthier way? Pick one and experiment this week with that.

Favorite food: _____

Remember that this is **YOUR** *Personal Journey with Food*. No one diet fits all. You have to get experience with food and learn what food works for you.

Want to Drive the Extra Mile?

If you are already familiar with whole foods and have already started incorporating them into your diet, why not go the extra mile?

The information below is useful to remember any time on your journey. Since we want to digest well in order to have more benefits from foods, we must take care of our digestive system and our gut flora.

Stress, poor nutrition, low moods, sleep problems, and some health conditions reduce our friendly gut flora population and may affect our body and mental health. If that happens, there is a condition that can develop called Leaky Gut Syndrome. It is believed that this syndrome is the first step in developing Psychology Syndromes and conditions like autism. Dr. Natasha Campbell-McBride states that all children are born with normal brains. However, if the gut flora does not develop correctly, the chance for autism increases as does the risk for other disorders such as attention deficit hyperactivity disorder, attention deficit disorder, dyslexia, or obsessive-compulsive disorder. She developed a diet protocol called the GAPSs diet. This diet focuses on detoxifying the body and restoring the gut flora. Dr. Campbell-McBride helped heal her son from autism, utilizing this protocol.

Leaky Gut Syndrome is a hyper-permeability of the tissue in the intestines. Large particles of food pass through the intestinal lining directly to the blood, causing the immune system to react and attack food proteins as if they were invaders. That's because the body "sees" them where they are not meant to be. It is believed that this process is the beginning of autoimmune diseases. Leaky gut can also be caused by taking medications in large amounts or for extended periods of time, by food allergies or food sensitivities, or by radiation therapy.

Choosing foods that nurture the microbiota will keep you on the right path in your journey. Add one or more items (if tolerated) from the following list to your diet each week to help the microbiota to thrive.

- Raw and fermented foods like Kimchi, Sauerkraut, and Tempeh
- Drinks like Kombucha and Water Kefir
- Bone broth
- Beans and legumes
- Whole grains
- Natural and sugarless Greek yogurt, Coconut yogurt, and Kefir
- Pre-biotic vegetable fiber (all kinds of greens)

Your Personal Journal With Food

Week Number:_____ Date:_____

What did you eat this week?

_____

_____

_____

_____

_____

How many glasses of plain water per day?_____
What did you do this week that makes you happy?

_____

_____

_____

This week, my percentage of processed food was: _____%
Whole Foods I tried this week and like:

_____

_____

_____

Favorite Food Experiment:

CHAPTER 5

_____

_____

_____

_____

_____

Time for an Alignment—
The Path of Mindfulness
By Tracy

"Thinking without awareness is the main
dilemma of human existence."

ECKHART TOLLE

What is mindfulness? Mindfulness is a primary and essential part of
your inner GPS.

Here is the Merriam-Webster definition.

Mindful

    The quality or state of being mindful

    *The practice of maintaining a nonjudgmental state of heightened
or complete awareness of one's thoughts, emotions, or experiences on a moment-to-moment basis; also: such a state of awareness*

    Mindful: aware of something that may be important

The following words are synonyms of mindfulness: Mindful, aware, present, conscious, attentive, heedful, observant, open-eyed, watchful, wide-awake.

Now that we know what mindfulness is, we can ask the question, what is the opposite of mindfulness? It is mindless.

I will again consult the Merriam-Webster dictionary.

Mindless

> A: *marked by a lack of mind or consciousness <a mindless sleep>*
> B(1): *marked by or displaying no use of the powers of the intellect<mindless violence> (2): requiring little attention or thought; especially: not intellectually challenging or stimulating <mindless work> <a mindless movie>*
> B: *not mindful: heedless <mindless of the consequences>*

The following words are synonyms of mindless: Careless, heedless, inattentive, incautious, unguarded, unheeding, unwary, unwise, illogical, irrational, untaught, unthinking, illogical, distracted.

Mindful? Mindless? Which word defines the way you eat? Which word represents the way you live? Are you mindful in some areas of your life, but completely absent (mindless) in others?

I lived my life mindlessly for a very long time. I was ignorant. I was unthinking. I was feeble-minded. I was like that in so many areas of my life. I was flying through the minutes, hours, days, weeks, months, and years without being fully present within the moment. If I was with my family, I was thinking about work. If I was eating lunch, I was thinking about work or that I needed to go exercise. If I was in a meeting, I was thinking about the work waiting for me at my desk. If I was driving, I was thinking about how I needed the traffic to go faster so I could be somewhere else. If I was exercising, I was thinking about work or grocery shopping, etc. When I ate, I ate fast and without any thought. I didn't care what I was putting in my mouth; into this body. My stress levels were through the roof. I couldn't focus on where I was or what I was doing. (This makes me think of Yoda's advice to Luke in the movie Star Wars. "This one a long time have I watched. All his life has he looked away, to the future, to the horizon. Never his mind on where he was, hmm? What he was doing. Hmm.")

Being a human being is a beautiful, yet complicated experience. We can visualize, plan, and strategize. We are able to remember the past and feel it all over again, as if it just happened. We can allow ourselves to live in the present and be wholly engaged in our lives.

For me, living in the present was very difficult to do. I always seemed to want to be somewhere else, or I believed I should be somewhere else. I prided myself on how I could think 5 to 10 steps ahead of my actions, thus allowing me to make good choices, or what I believed at the time were good choices. I prided myself on being able to look at the past as a learning lesson. But sometimes, my vision of the future and my thoughts of the past brought a feeling of terrible anxiety. I had a hard time being present and comfortable with "me" during the present moment. This caused me much grief and distress on a daily basis.

Because being present and mindful in life was challenging for me, my relationships with others and with food suffered. But as I began to live more mindfully, my suffering diminished tremendously! And because it was a challenge for me, I know that mindful living may also be a challenge for you. You can begin being mindful in your life by being aware of how your thoughts, your lifestyle, and your habits help to determine everything you do. Mindful living begins with mindful thoughts and behavior, from what you eat, how you take care of your body, your home, and pets, how you relate in your relationships, and how you approach spirituality.

I recently read an article in our local, Seattle Times, "New Strategy, Ancient Tool. Military Turns to Mindfulness Training." With the military finally turning to mindfulness to help their soldiers excel, maybe that's a sign that it would be good for you too. When we are mindful, we remember things better. We can be more intentional. Our abilities in many areas can improve. We can also manage current and past stressors/ traumas much better. It helps the mind adapt to changing environments and circumstances.

With this in mind, are you aware of your thoughts and where your focus tends to be? It is imperative to know that what we think about, our mind has the power to bring into our lives. As you go about your day, stop every now and to think about how you're feeling, and what your thoughts are at that moment. Are you feeling joyful? Positive? Anguished? Grateful? Resentful? Hateful? Victimized? Are your thoughts judgmental? Authentic to you? Self-trusting? A bit paranoid? Supportive? Purposeful? Is your gut, your intuition speaking to you, and are you listening? Take a moment to jot down how you are feeling right now and where your thoughts are.

_____

_____

_____

_____

_____

Did you know that our subconscious is not aware of what is real and what is not real? Whatever we can imagine, our subconscious believes to be true. Our thoughts are a guidance system for our subconscious to act upon and believe me; the subconscious does act upon them. If our thoughts are chronically negative, we will attract and live life from that negative mindset. If our thoughts are consistently positive, purposeful, and loving, we will attract and live life from that mindset. With that said, we shouldn't despair if we have negative thoughts now and then or have a bad day. As humans, we are going to have these thoughts and feelings. I am talking about consistent and chronic negative thoughts. Take note and be mindful of where your thoughts drift. Ask yourself when you notice them, "How is this serving me, and is it warranted?"

So, what does this have to do with food and dieting? Your thoughts and your mood can dictate what you eat. And what you eat will influence your mood and actions. Your food, your mood, your thoughts, and your actions are all directly connected and influence one another!

Once you see how your mood, thoughts, and feelings influence the foods you choose to eat and how the foods you choose to eat influence your thoughts, moods, and feelings, then you will begin to see what changes you need to make. That is the place in this whole process where you will know exactly where you are in your journey. It is your starting point. Mindfulness is the key skill that allows you to begin and then move through this process. Practicing mindfulness will help you to take the supportive steps you need to take every day and to learn what works for your body and your life. It can mean meeting the real YOU for the first time!

In my journey to get to where I am now, there was a time when I never paid attention to how food made me feel, nor did I understand how it was serving me—good or bad. And I never acknowledged to myself how I used it emotionally.

Answer the following questions as honestly as you can.

How would you rate your relationship with food?

_____

_____

_____

_____

_____

Is it balanced? Are you able to make healthy choices consistently?

_____

_____

_____

_____

_____

Do you feel confident in what foods are healthy for you?

_____

_____

_____

_____

_____

Are you addicted to foods that you know are hurting you but feel you have no power to stop eating them? If so, which?

_____

_____

_____

_____

_____

Do you eat healthily, but do you find it stressful and extreme?

_____

_____

_____

_____

_____

Is your relationship with food one where you have control, or does it control you?

_____

_____

_____

_____

_____

Do you have a solid understanding of what "food" is and what it is indeed for?

_____

_____

_____

_____

Does your relationship with food make you sad and distressed, or does it empower you?

_____

_____

_____

_____

What did food mean to you as an adolescent child?

_____

_____

_____

_____

_____

As a teenager?

_____

_____

_____

_____

_____

As an adult?

_____

_____

_____

_____

_____

Were you able to answer these questions with confidence? Did you feel any anxiety as you answered any of them? Were you indifferent? Did you feel unsure? Did you hold judgment against yourself? I felt so many different things when I answered these for myself years ago.

Becoming "mindful" about food is one of the most empowering skills you can learn. Learning this practice has given me the ability to make healthy and supportive choices, maintain a healthy weight, avoid bloating, and to finally let go of the Yo-Yo diet lifestyle.

Being mindful of the food I eat has also enabled me to utilize a gift we all have: The gift to honestly hear and understand the signals our body gives to us every time we eat. My body sent me signals that I ignored for the majority of my life. I didn't hear or understand them until I began practicing mindfulness. Mindfulness enabled me to listen and hear the signals my body was sending me. Then, I chose to act upon them. If I had been able to listen and learn at a much earlier age, it would have alleviated my constant weight issues as well as many of the anxiety challenges I faced growing up and in my earlier adult life.

Although the tools we are using are the same, your path may very well be different than mine was. Your relationship with food is yours and yours alone. No one else lives in your space. You need to walk *Your Personal Journey with Food* and figure out what makes your body feel its best. Be curious, learn all you can, and honor your body's signals.

Let's move forward so that you can begin to discover your personal relationship with food.

To do this, you will start to eat "mindfully." You can eat mindfully anytime and anywhere. Others around you don't even have to know that you are doing it. (However, if you can teach this practice to others, imagine what a positive impact it will have on your family and friends!)

The following is an exercise you can do at your very next meal or snack. I chose to write this exercise with a scenario that involved friends. As Ingrid states in **Chapter 1, Before You Start Your Journey**, we are social creatures, and food is a significant part of our social experience.

Exercise: Mindful Eating—Dining Out with Friends

- ⊕ When arriving at the restaurant, take note of your surroundings and others.
- ⊕ Restaurant: Notice scents, temperature, colors, busy, slow, hectic, clean, dirty.
- ⊕ Guests at the table: What are they wearing? Are their eyes alive or distant? What is their posture? What is yours? What is the mood of each person? What energy do you feel coming from them? What energy are you giving off to them?
- ⊕ Table setting: Take note of the silverware, plates, is there something visually pleasing to you at the table? A candle? A flower? Nothing?
- ⊕ The menu: What types of food does the restaurant serve?

Of the choices, which ones speak to you the most. Notice what happens to you physically when you read the menu. Do you react differently to different items? Do any of them make your mouth start to water, and your stomach gurgle with excitement? Do others make you say, "Ick! I would never eat that!" Do you tend to gravitate towards a particular type of food? Take note of that, as it is a significant clue. (I recommend you write this in your journal.) Consider what you are going to order, thus put into your body. Is it something you want to absorb and have become part of you?

⊕ Conversation: After you have ordered, continue paying attention to your reactions to the environment and those at the table. Are you stressed, rushed? Are you calm and relaxed? Are you listening to others speak, or do you think about something else instead? These things will determine how your body will be able to digest what you are about to eat. Do your best to relax and help your body prepare for digestion.

⊕ Eating: When your food arrives, be grateful and thank your server for bringing it to you.

⊕ Now you get to start eating mindfully.

⊕ How does the food look on the plate? Does the meal seem oversized? Do you have any thoughts about it being too much or too little? Do you think the portion sizes are right for you personally? What colors do you see? What effort do you imagine went into the preparation, and where do you think all the ingredients came from to make you this meal? We tend to lose sight of these things. Who grew the lettuce? Where was it grown? If you are eating meat, where do you think it came from and was that animal treated fairly? Again, consider what you are going to put into your body. Is it something you want to absorb and have become part of you?

⊕ Now breathe in the aroma of your food. Can you detect the different spices? Can you discern the scent of the main course versus the side dishes?

⊕ As you do this, notice how your body is reacting. Are you getting good signals, bad signals, or indifferent signals? Is your mouth watering?

⊕ Choose the correct utensil required to eat your meal. Cut your first bite and bring it to your mouth. Notice the various textures of color and scent. Imagine what this food is going to taste like and then place it in your mouth. Put down your eating utensils.

⊕ What does it feel like as you begin to chew? What are the different textures, and what are the different underlying flavors? You will be compelled to swallow but don't. Keep chewing as long as you possibly can. Let every single taste-bud get in on the action. Allow yourself the opportunity to TASTE your food completely! Chewing will allow you to get all the pleasure and flavor of each bite. As you chew, notice how this changes the flavor of your food and how your saliva is helping to break it down. Chew as much as possible before swallowing. Try to chew each bite at least 30 times. (Yes, this will be a challenge! We are a society of 3 to 5 chews per bite!) I promise it gets easier with practice. And I promise you will feel so much better when you chew your food thoroughly.

⊕ To learn more about chewing and why it is so important for your overall digestion and health, be sure to download your free pdf at **www.journeywithfood.com.**

⊕ With each bite, repeat the same process. Pick up your eating utensils, place the food in your mouth, then put down your utensils. Use your eyes, your sense of smell, your taste buds, pay attention to textures, and chew, chew, chew.

⊕ Throughout your meal, pay attention to your relationship with the food you are eating. Ask yourself as you are eating, is this food going to give my body the right nutrients to function as best it can or is it going to harm my body? Do I even know the answer to that question? Am I getting full?

How is my stomach responding to this meal? Do I feel good, or is my stomach painfully full or bloated? If painfully full or bloated, how quickly did this happen? Do I really like the taste of this meal? Do you experience any other sensations?

⊕ Feeling Full: When you START to feel full, STOP EAT-ING. Call your server over and have your leftovers wrapped up to take with you. Do not eat past the signal that you are full. Listen to your body and fight the urge to force food into your stomach. When you begin to eat this way, you may need to call your server over quickly because you may not be able to stop eating. Do not look at this as "loss," but be excited that you get to enjoy the remainder of your meal at a later time. Be proud that you noticed you were getting full.

⊕ To learn more about portion sizes specific to you, be sure to download your free pdf at **www.journeywithfood.com**.

⊕ Finishing Up: When finished, take a deep breath through your nose and let it out gently through a relaxed mouth. Be grateful for the opportunity to experience your meal and for the time with your friends.

Mindful eating allows you to learn a great deal about yourself, your body, and about others. When you practice this skill, you will have the ability to unmask foods that do not serve. You can control your weight because you now pay attention to when you are getting full, and you do not mindlessly push your stomach to accept food after it is full. You will chew your food adequately so that the nutrients from that food are more readily available for digestion. When we eat fast, we never give our bodies the chance to tell us we are full until it is too late. We also don't give our body time to prepare for digestion. By eating slowly and mindfully, you will uncover foods that could be making you feel sick or sluggish and tired.

Remember to pay attention to how you feel before a meal. Are you rushed? Are you stressed? Are you craving a particular food? Are you really hungry or just bored? What are you craving, and do you really know what that craving is trying to tell you? Be sure to acknowledge how you feel during and after your meal. Your body will be talking to you for hours, even days after a meal. Keep listening!

When you eat mindfully at home you can incorporate all that I have noted above, but add the following:

⊕ Set the table nicely. Use your favorite dishes and utensils. Make the table pleasing. Remove all clutter.

⊕ While preparing your meal, do so in a calm fashion. Realize you are cooking something that will be nourishing your body as well as those dining with you. Read all the labels and be aware of all the ingredients. Do they pass your inspection?

⊕ Enjoy the colors, the textures, and the scents of all the different ingredients.

⊕ Turn off the TV. Go ahead and just have silence or feel free to play pleasing music in the background.

⊕ Teach those dining with you this concept and let everyone participate together. Help to make it a fun and insightful experience for all.

Living Mindfully

This practice is very similar to the method of mindful eating. They are integrated. You cannot have one without the other.

Being aware of your thoughts, surroundings, relationships, and body signals on a daily basis will help you sculpt the life that you desire. The majority of our world is so fast-paced. Information is coming at us from all angles. Many of us do not know how to be at peace or how to stop the noise. We have lost the skill.

When you become mindful in life, you then step into real purpose and strength.

Let me say this—no one is perfect, and I don't believe it is possible to be mindful every moment of every day. This book is not about anyone being "perfect." Just realize that the mind likes to wander off; as some folks say, "squirrel!" It takes practice to keep the mind on task and in the present moment. Because of this, it is important to catch yourself when you aren't living in the present and bring your mind back to the current task at hand and settle in.

For example, I never realized how nervous and anxious I was while watching standard TV. The audio, the commercial volume ringing is louder than the TV show, the violence, etc. I get impatient and frustrated. By noticing my reactions when watching TV, I was practicing mindfulness. Knowing this now, I minimize my TV viewing.

As we learn to eat our food mindfully and honor our body by listening to it before, during, and after we eat, we can also learn to do the same with our daily activities and relationships by acknowledging the signals we receive intuitively. Knowing your values and priorities will help you to live in integrity with yourself and others.

One way to help make this part of mindfulness a reality in life is to find the root cause of your emotions. Notice what makes you feel happy, sad, distressed, strong, courageous, loving. But remember, there is no judgment when you notice things about yourself; you are only looking to find out where you are. If you are not sure of where you are, how can you even begin the journey to where you want to be? I understand that this discovery can be a bit painful. But it is also very freeing!

As with mindful eating, living mindfully is a process. But because everyone is different, the starting points and the journey will be different for each person.

We are now at the end of this chapter. Please, take a moment and go back to the **Introduction** and review your **Feet on the Pavement View** questionnaire, and your **Life Radar**. Take a moment to review how you scored yourself in all categories.

If you see any areas in which you need to improve, it's OK. Each area is connected, and as you start working on one area of your life, many of the same disciplines needed to improve in that area, are the same disciplines required to improve in all the other areas. Mindfulness is a crucial one.

Are you feeling overwhelmed and uncertain? Know that even a coach needs a coach, and it can be constructive for you to utilize one as well. A coach can help you prioritize each area and help you use mindfulness to establish a plan. Want help with building your program? Feel free to reach out to us; we would love to hear from you!

Email us at **start@journeywithfood.com**

Your Personal Journal With Food

Week Number:_____ Date:_____

What did you eat this week?

_____

_____

_____

_____

_____

How many glasses of plain water per day? _____
What did you do this week that makes you happy?

_____

_____

Were you able to identify your feelings and emotional states when
you were eating?

_____

_____

This week, my percentage of processed food was: _____
Whole Foods I tried this week and liked:

_____

_____

Healthier versions of Favorite Food Experiment:

_____

_____

Number of mindful meals this week:_____

Mindful Exercise for the Week:

With your camera take pictures of every plate of food you eat, snacks and meals.

Also take a picture of your environment, no matter if you are at the table or in your car.

Do this for a week.

Do not hide anything.

Commit to being an investigator and learn about your behaviors related to food.

At the end of each day, review your pictures and write in your journal how you feel in regards to what you ate.

As you do this, can you associate any of the foods to sensations or any symptom?

If you need some help understanding what a symptom may be, feel free to utilize the list of symptoms in **Chapter 6, Your Journey Buddies—Symptoms As A Co-pilot** as your compass.

CHAPTER 6

Your Journey Buddies— Symptoms as a Co-Pilot

By Ingrid and Tracy

Once you start your journey with food, your body will be your co-pilot. By listening to your body, you will know if you are on the right track. Your body will speak using signals, usually known as "symptoms and cravings." I encourage you to appreciate these messages instead of feeling a victim of them. You are not your symptoms; your cravings do not control you, and they do not define you. With a thankful attitude, your cravings and symptoms will guide you to a better place.

Let the "judge" feeling and all those thoughts that deplete you exit your car. Invite only the mindset and feelings that encourage you to move forward with you on your trip.

With an open mind, curiosity, and self-love, your body will "speak," and you will listen.

Symptoms

I would like to share my journey with you. It started when I was a baby, with my body rejecting almost every healthy nutrition source, even breast milk. Instead, I survived by drinking powdered milk formula. When I was a kid, most vegetables, leafy greens, fruits, milk, fish, and eggs gave me nausea, causing me to vomit. Lunch and dinner were torture for me. I was forced to eat meat and didn't like legumes or rice, but fried food, sugary food, and things made with flour such as pasta: I just loved those! My favorite foods were cookies, cakes, sodas, and "juices" made from some syrup with brilliant colors that tasted more like chewing gum than fruit.

My body and personality soon changed from a very skinny and active kid to a shy and overweight girl who felt terrible about herself. I was ashamed of being so "big." At 14 years old, I was able to lose weight in a not recommended way: hepatitis! I possibly ate some contaminated food, plus having a very weak and toxic liver (for all my unhealthy food choices), which resulted in one month in bed without chocolate and fried food. That was the first time I was forced to listen to my body. Before that, all the signals my body was giving me (trying to tell me my nutrition was wrong) I thought were normal: constipation, heartburn, skin rashes, cavities, and urinary tract infections. Thanks to hepatitis, my cravings for fried food reduced dramatically, and I started to eat some vegetables in soups.

When I moved to Chile, I can say that I ate a little bit better, but my diet was mostly inflammatory and consisted of junk food. I was living on my own, facing the chore of trying to nurture myself while my fridge was full of frozen, microwavable food. My pantry had only packaged and processed food in it. The "just add water, and magically it will turn into something you can eat" kind. Several days in a row, I ate boxed cereals for breakfast, lunch, and dinner. I did this because cereal was easy to prepare. Plus, the label stated it had almost all the vitamins and minerals I needed.

At 20 years of age (while I still had teenage acne), I started to get wrinkles. My weight was increasing. I felt so tired. I could not run continuously for a single block. If I had to use stairs, I was breathless on the second floor. Bad circulation, heartburn, constipation, terrible back pain, infections in my lungs, sinusitis and urinary infections were regular occurrences.

At 28, I started getting severe pain in my kidney area every spring. Each year I ended up in the emergency room with no precise diagnosis. The doctors said I could have kidney stones, but they never found any. My bodyweight was between 85 and 88 kilos (185 to 195 pounds). The fat tissue in my body was at 45%, yet I was malnourished. Slowly, I started to improve my food habits. I traded the one liter per day of soda for plain water. I also started walking for one and a half hours every day. After just one month, I had lost 10 kilos (22 pounds) by only incorporating those two things.

Years later, after reading about Integrative Nutrition and doing emotional healing therapies, I learned that the kidney symptoms I suffered from were related to bad food choices and emotional repression. I was intoxicated from eating too much sugar, flavor additives, color additives, fried food, as well as from silenced and suppressed emotions.

I learned to eat fruits and vegetables, and while I was improving on that, I let go of the unhealthy stuff: unhealthy food, bad relationships, negative beliefs, and unhealthy habits that were poisoning my body, my heart, and my soul.

Now, I understand that I was always hungry due to being nutritionally starved as well as emotionally empty. These voids would never be filled by eating the foods that I had been eating for most of my life. I was eating the same things over and over again.

- 7 am boxed cereal with yogurt or toast with butter
- 9 am a cheese sandwich
- 11 am cookies
- 1 pm pasta with salad
- 4 pm cookies
- 7 pm chicken and lettuce wrap

Do you notice a pattern in my choices of food? I was eating flour all day long. After I realized the pattern I was in, I was able to make changes that alleviated all the symptoms that had been "normal" for me. This example of the pattern of my choices of food shows why mindfulness is key to *Your Personal Journey with Food*. Tracy will guide you on how to start a mindful life in **Chapter 5, Time for an Alignment—The Path of Mindfulness.**

As I progressed on my journey, I followed a 10-day detox plan, which consisted of an 80% raw vegan diet along with some colonic therapy. After that, I had finally detoxed and nourished myself. Since then, I have not felt the kidney pain again. And not only that, my skin has become more brilliant. Now at 40 years old with a 1-year-old baby, I have more energy than in my 20s! I keep myself in better physical condition, and I have been able to maintain a healthy weight without dieting. Thanks to the signals my body was sending me, my symptoms of illness, I could find the path to feeling better. I am sure you can do that, too.

Symptoms are the way your body speaks to you. Those symptoms are not you, nor are they because of your age or because of your genetics. They are evidence that something is going on, something you need to attend to. By choosing exercise, better sleeping habits, and improving your food choices, your body will begin to speak to you in other, better ways.

In some cases, it is imperative to see a doctor and take medication. But please don´t use a doctor's diagnosis to surrender to any symptoms you might have. A diagnosis is not an excuse to avoid going on a healthy food journey. I am sad to see that some people will view a diagnosis as a cast-iron truth, and there is nothing that can be done but to live a life filled with medications. That isn't true.

Chronic health issues such as type II diabetes, insulin resistance, high cholesterol levels, or obesity are usually symptoms of unhealthy food choices, poor sleep, and a sedentary lifestyle. To be truly healthy, you want to address the cause of the diagnosis, not just the symptoms. So, why not begin taking steps to improve those habits?

When I met Tracy, her history with food was inspiring to me. We met via a Skype call to complete a homework assignment for school at The Institute for Integrative Nutrition, and on my screen, this stunning woman appeared. She was ten years older than me, but she looked younger than me!

When she told me that she changed her insulin resistance diagnosis by choosing better food, I felt that we needed to tell every single soul in the world about how the food that is on our plates impacts our health and our life.

Tracy, could you please share how your symptoms helped you build a better relationship with food?

"Absolutely! I had been a "yo-yo" dieter since my high school years. Food was my comfort, as well as my nemesis. You see, I saw myself as never being "good enough." I felt unworthy. I was not perfect, like other people. I was far from deserving of my life's dreams. It was always someone else's turn before mine. "Don't shine too brightly, Tracy," I would think to myself," who are you to be anything." It was a constant inner struggle that I didn't understand as an adult, let alone as a child, that was always tormenting me.

I know today that my diet actually triggered many of my emotional challenges. My diet was also making me physically sick. My diet would make my stomach hurt, and my heart race, thus giving me feelings of anxiety and distress. My diet was wreaking havoc on my body and mind.

I would have a meal, then feel sick. I would then try to eat something else in an attempt to feel better. It became a vicious cycle: gaining weight, dieting, gaining weight, then dieting again. I thought it was normal to feel this way and that there was nothing I could do, so I just accepted it.

As a child, before bed, I would have a nice warm glass of milk and sugar toast. Some nights, I had homemade buttered popcorn or cheese popcorn. The theory was not to send me to bed hungry, so a snack was always welcome! For breakfast, my mother would want me to have a healthy breakfast. The usual options were oatmeal and milk, or toast, eggs, and milk. I now know that oatmeal, eggs, and milk, although deemed healthy for most people, were the main reason I felt so awful. It turns out that I have a high sensitivity to dairy, oats, sugar cane, and eggs! With this meal plan, I would wake up in the morning feeling lethargic and nauseous from the milk and popcorn the night before. Then, I was off to school, still feeling nauseous and anxious from not only my night-time snack hangover but my breakfast. I dreaded eating breakfast!

In grade school, I recall going to school feeling anxious and ill, getting diarrhea, being sent to the office with terrible stomach cramps, and being sent home. This episode happened often, and it was thought that I just had separation anxiety and that I would grow out of it. It was the mid-1970's and not much was understood about food sensitivities and how they could cause the symptoms I was having.

I carried these misunderstood food sensitivities and symptoms with me into my mid-40's. Eating and feeling sick. Eating and feeling "fat" immediately. Eating and having my stomach literally ache and bulge out, making my waistband tight and uncomfortable. I thought this was just feeling full. I didn't understand that what I was feeling was actually "bloating." There is a big difference between bloating and being full. Have you ever eaten something and been full within just a couple of bites? If so, you could be "bloating" from that food.

In my early 40's, I got a big wake-up call. I had a great deal of stress in my life at that time; a knee injury that was not healing as hoped, long hours at work, no exercise, too much wine, and chocolate; the perfect storm. I was thirty or more pounds over-weight, unhappy, and felt like giving up. (I couldn't bear to weigh myself.) I recall wishing I had appreciated my body a long time ago instead of hating it. I bought into the "everyone has this happen as they age" mentality. Over time I started to notice that I was often very thirsty and always having to run to the restroom. It was definitely a different "kind" of thirst and definitely a different kind of "potty-urge." When I went in for my annual physical, my doctor notified me that my blood sugar levels were high. I was on my way to becoming a type 2 diabetic. My doctor told me that I could change this with diet. I saw this as a statement of hope.

I didn't want to go on yet another "diet." I was tired of dieting, and I didn't want to feel deprived. I decided this didn't matter. I had to change. My first assignment was minimizing my sugar intake and eliminating refined carbohydrates. I was to switch from refined grains to whole grains. No problem, right? Not so fast. At home, I had a big pantry full of beautiful white flour, various breakfast cereals, potato chips, tortilla chips, yummy white penne pasta and white linguine noodles, instant baking mixes, popcorn, white rice, bread, cookies, fruit snacks, crackers, pretzels, etc. I also had two teenagers and a husband at home that liked ALL of those wonderful "foods!" I remember talking with my family and telling them that I could not eat those foods any longer. In a way, it was a big relief as most of them always made me feel sick anyway. Now I could say "no" when offered these foods.

I started my new life by eliminating bread and pasta. Giving up pasta was very challenging for me. I absolutely LOVED a delicious al dente pasta noodle smothered with a zesty red marinara or a creamy Alfredo chicken mushroom sauce. Top it off with fresh parmesan cheese, and I was a happy camper.

Although unsure, I started integrating whole grain pasta with my white pasta. By doing this, my transition was more manageable for my taste buds to accept. Since then, I have substituted whole grain pasta with spaghetti squash, zucchini noodles, or cauliflower and have grain pasta only a few times a year. I utilized this process with other foods, as well. Making changes and allowing my taste buds to learn to like something new. I basically "crowded out" the foods that were harming my body with those that supported it and helped it heal.

As time progressed, I began to pay attention to how I felt before, during, and after I ate. I finally understood that I did not have to feel sick all the time. I learned to eat "mindfully." If I began to feel ill during or after a meal, I made a mental note of that food and did my best not to eat it again. (I still do this now.) I stopped eating eggs and most dairy. After some time had passed, I went ahead and had a food sensitivity panel done. It was an exciting moment for me as it affirmed that yes, I have a high sensitivity to egg, specifically egg whites, milk, soft cheeses, oats, and pineapple. What a relief it was to know my body had been telling me this all of my life. There had been a real reason for my symptoms. I wasn't "crazy" after all. (Sometimes I felt I was!)

One of the best things you can do for your well-being is to pay attention to your symptoms, listen to your body, and respect what it is telling you. Paying attention to my symptoms and then modifying my lifestyle to eliminate them, has been my biggest lesson. By doing this, I have succeeded in changing my health. I now "hear" my body. I respect what it is telling me.

As Tracy has illustrated so well, listening to your symptoms is key to finding ways to improve them. It is probably a good time to say again that symptoms are the body's way of telling us that something is not working. But those symptoms do NOT define you.

There are symptoms related to poor health habits, food sensitivities, nutritional deficiencies/toxicities, or unhealthy food. We created a list of them in the assessment questionnaire in the **Introduction**. This list is not equal to a medical diagnosis or treatment and will not guarantee a disease cure. Please review this list. My intention is to ask you if you have any of the listed symptoms and could they be related to the way you eat and your lifestyle habits.

Cravings

Do cravings take control of your steering wheel? How many times did you stop your diet because of an irresistible craving? Why do we even have cravings?

Multiple factors could lead us to crave something. Below is a list of the source of cravings that Tracy and I see most frequently in our work with clients.

⊕ Nutritional imbalances: If your body needs some kind of nutrient, it can let you know in the form of a craving.

⊕ Dehydration: Sometimes, the thirst signal can be confused with the hungry signal.

⊕ Eating too much salt or too much sugar: If you are eating something very salty, your body may need to balance that flavor with something sugary or vice versa.

⊕ Hormonal imbalances: Some people feel cravings due to hormonal imbalances, for example, chocolate during the menstrual cycle. This particular craving is tied with nutritional craving because a woman in her cycle loses some nutrients (magnesium, for example) found in chocolate. Plus, cacao increases serotonin levels (as we saw in **Chapter 1, Before You Start Your Journey**) and creates a comfortable feeling.

⊕ Habits: Perhaps you associate a behavior with a particular craving, for example, having dessert after every meal. The point is to notice if you are eating because of behavior or because you are hungry.

⊕ Emotional cravings: eating because you feel something, and you want to comfort or reward yourself somehow instead of examining that emotion.

⊕ Cultural cravings or DNA cravings: When you want to eat something that connects you with your culture or your heritage.

Now that we know where it comes from, what should you do when you have a craving? Keep in mind that eating a variety of whole foods and staying hydrated will reduce many of your cravings. (The first three bullets on the list.) But if you are eating healthy and still craving something, try this:

1. Drink a glass of water (just in case).
2. Connect with your emotions. Is this craving due to some-

thing you are feeling? If so, take a break, breathe, and try to solve what is bringing that emotion.

3. If it is not emotional or if you still want to eat that special thing, replace it with a healthier version.

4. If none of the previous ideas work: give yourself permission to satisfy your craving but do it mindfully: stick to one serving and take your time to enjoy the flavor. Do this only sparingly.

Exercise: Knowing Your Journey Buddies

This week, with your camera, take photos of every plate of food you eat. Take pictures of the things you snack on as well. Do this for a week. Do not hide anything. Commit to being an investigator and learning about not only any symptoms you may have regarding your food, but your behaviors related to food. At the end of each day, review your pictures and do a thoughtful analysis of your body and mind. If you have any symptoms, be sure to list them. Rate your symptoms on a scale of intensity. A '0' would signify no symptom, and '10' would signify a severe symptom.

Ask Yourself These Questions

Is your food healthy?
How can you add one or two whole foods?
Is there a food you are eating too much of?
Can you add some variety?

Make some healthy changes to your meal plan and review the symptoms again in 15 days.

Keep in mind that acknowledging your symptoms is a critical part of *Your Personal Journey with Food*. It is an empowering process that will have a positive impact on your life. It is a self-loving tool and a road to walk every day.

	Symptom(s) Intensity Start Date	Changes to Introduce	Symptom(s) Intensity After 15 days
Mon			
Tue			
Wed			
Thu			
Fri			
Sat			
Sun			

Your Personal Journal With Food

Week Number:_____ Date:_____

What did you eat this week?

_____

_____

_____

_____

_____

How many glasses of plain water per day?_____
What did you do this week that makes you happy?

_____

_____

Did you have any symptoms related to food this week?

_____

_____

If you do, rate those symptoms on a scale of intensity.

_____

_____

Review the intensity of those symptoms in 15 days. What did you find?

_____

_____

Can you add more variety to your meals?_____

Percentage of processed foods this week:_____

Percentage of Mindful meals this week:_____

CHAPTER 7

Picking the Right Fuel— Food Sensitivities

By Tracy

The healthiest and nutritionally packed food can be one of the most devastating and unhealthy foods to eat if you are intolerant, sensitive, or allergic to it. Here's a way to think of it. You pull up to the gas station because you need to fill your gas tank. The pump you pull up to has several different fuel options. Here in the United States, we generally see unleaded gas. The octane levels are; Regular 87, midgrade 88-90, and premium at 91-94. We also have diesel fuel at our gas stations. Which fuel should you pick for your car? You could consult your owner's manual, and it will tell you. Or most vehicles have the fuel requirements listed near the gas cap. Because you're tired and not paying attention, you accidentally put diesel fuel in your car, which was only supposed to take premium unleaded gas. Technically, there is nothing wrong with diesel fuel. BUT there is a problem when it is fueling an engine that needs premium unleaded fuel. Your car's engine is not going to run well at all, and you will most likely have a costly mechanic bill that arises because of your error.

Having a food sensitivity or allergy is a similar concept. There may not be anything wrong with the food you ate, in itself. And that food may work perfectly for someone else, but for you…. it does not work at all. Having a sensitivity or allergy to a particular food can wreak havoc on your body as well as your emotions. Sometimes the body's response is immediate when we consume something it doesn't like. Sometimes the reaction can take several days or be almost unnoticeable. One thing that is becoming clearer and clearer is that by continuing to subject your body to foods that you are sensitive to can cause your body harm.

It can be a little confusing to know the difference between a food intolerance/sensitivity and a food allergy. Food sensitivity and allergy are two different things. A food allergy happens when your body mistakenly attacks food proteins as if they are harmful germs or viruses. This reaction can be anywhere from a nuisance to a dangerous, life-threatening anaphylactic reaction. An allergic reaction will usually show itself within minutes to several hours after eating the suspect food. If you are allergic to a particular food, you could have any of the various symptoms listed below. For more detailed information, I recommend visiting the Food Allergy Research and Education website at www.foodallergy.org/sypmptoms.

Symptoms

- ⊕ Hives
- ⊕ Eczema
- ⊕ Redness of the skin around eyes
- ⊕ Itchy mouth or ear canal
- ⊕ Nausea or vomiting
- ⊕ Diarrhea
- ⊕ Stomach pain
- ⊕ Nasal congestion or a runny nose
- ⊕ Sneezing
- ⊕ Slight, dry cough

- Odd taste in the mouth
- Uterine contractions

Severe Symptoms

- Obstructive swelling of the lips, tongue and or throat
- Trouble swallowing
- Shortness of breath or wheezing
- Turning blue
- A drop in blood pressure (feeling faint, confused, weak, passing out)
- Loss of consciousness
- Chest pain
- A weak or "thread" pulse
- The sense of "impending doom"

A food sensitivity, on the other hand, does not cause an immune response, as stated above. However, it can cause discomfort and inflammation in the body. Symptoms can be immediate or may not show up for days after you eat the offending food.

Symptoms of food intolerance may include any of the following:

- Bloating
- Diarrhea
- Constipation
- Stomach cramps
- Gas
- Eczema
- Increased Heart Rate
- Swelling

If you are experiencing any of these symptoms, it's time to put on your super-sleuth hat and begin your investigation. I promise you; it is worth figuring these things out.

Because I didn't understand what "bloating" was until six or so years ago, I thought I would offer up a description of it for others who are unsure. You see, I thought I was "full" when, in fact, I was bloated. I recall looking at myself in the mirror sideways after a meal and noticed that my abdomen would literally be distended several inches. Bloating happened to me fairly quickly and had for most of my life, so I didn't know any different. It happened (and still does happen) if I eat cheese, certain kinds of bread, oats, drink beer or wine. It was also painful. I also noticed that when I ate one or two pieces of soft cheese, I would be uncomfortably "full" within minutes. This symptom is NOT "full." This symptom is bloating.

Have you been experiencing bloating and thought you were just full? Does your abdomen painfully expand even if you haven't eaten too large a serving? If so, this is bloating. Do you suspect you may have a food allergy or sensitivity? As I stated earlier, consuming foods that your body is sensitive to can make you feel awful as well as cause damage to cells in your body.

A challenging aspect of food sensitivity and allergy is that they can develop and change over time. Symptoms can also vary, making it a frustrating process to isolate.

Most of my life, I have felt fatigued, bloated (fat), and nauseated. I didn't know any different or think to ask about it because I figured it was normal. As I explain in **Chapter 6, Your Journey Buddies, Symptoms as a Co-Pilot**, I had a high level of anxiety along with tummy issues. I recall my diet as a child, and although it technically consisted of healthy food, it was, in fact, not always healthy for me.

Often when I went to school feeling sick, I usually had had oatmeal with milk for breakfast. I would end up in the nurse's office with severe stomach cramps and diarrhea issues then sent home. Of course, a few hours later, I felt just fine. The next day, tummy issues, sent home, felt better, etc. Therefore, it was assumed that I just had anxiety due to being at school. I believe I had anxiety because I was so afraid that I wouldn't make it to the bathroom in time!

In the mid-'70s, food was not looked at as a possible cause of my symptoms. (In fact, today this is still an issue.) Therefore, my breakfast was overlooked as a potential catalyst for my stomach and intestinal problems. At night, we usually always had popcorn with butter and cheese on it with a glass of milk, or mom would make us a yummy piece of toast and warm milk, so we weren't hungry. I'd wake up in the morning feeling lethargic and a bit under the weather every day. I know now that oatmeal and dairy are high triggers for me and make me feel sick every time I have them.

Food sensitivities and food allergies can be a challenge to isolate because you cannot necessarily test them with a skin prick test. You can, however, test for food sensitivities and allergies through elimination diets as well as through blood tests. As with most advice relating to foods and wellness, there is much debate over the best way to find out if you are sensitive to a particular food or ingredient.

We will look at both elimination diets and blood tests, and you can decide which one is best for you. Here is an example of an elimination diet.

Elimination Diet—3 Weeks to 90 Days

- ⊕ Begin to remove processed foods by crowding out with whole foods
- ⊕ Remove possible food allergy suspects such as eggs, corn, shellfish, dairy, gluten, peanuts, yeast, soy
- ⊕ Remove irritants to the gut such as alcohol, caffeine, sodas, "sugar-free" products, "gum" additives such as guar, Arabic, carrageenan
- ⊕ Take a probiotic (I recommend to my clients that they should take a probiotic every day even when not on a special elimination diet.)
- ⊕ Track how you feel during the prescribed time and note any changes you experience. This is an excellent time to utilize your new mindfulness skills. (If you haven't read **Chapter**

5, Time for an Alignment—The Path of Mindfulness yet, do so before you begin the elimination diet.)

⊕ After your elimination time is over, pick one food to add back in and pay attention to how your body reacts. (This is when you want to incorporate your "super sleuth" skills. Become a detective and listen, feel, observe.)

When you begin eating the selected item again, pay attention, and ask yourself these questions:

⊕ How do I feel during my meal?

⊕ How do I feel after my meal?

⊕ Do any symptoms occur within three days of eating this item again?

⊕ Do the symptoms occur on three separate occasions of eating that food?

If your body still reacts poorly, remove that food item again. If not, consider keeping it in your diet regimen. Continue this process with all the foods you initially removed. Does this process seem daunting? If so, the next option may be better for you.

Blood Tests

There are several blood tests available today to aid you in discovering any food sensitivities or food allergies you might have:

The first test is the ALCAT, which stands for the Antigen Leukocyte Antibody Test. This blood test not only tests for foods you are sensitive to, but it can also check for chemical and mold sensitivities.

The second test is the IgG Food Antibody Assessment—Immunoglobulin G Test. This test looks for sensitivities and measures IgG antibody levels to 87 foods.

You can get this test done by most Naturopathic and Integrative doctors.

You can also order your own IgG Food Sensitivity Panel from Your Labwork.

The URL is https://yourlabwork.com/?ref=489. (Be aware that this link is a customized affiliate link created for *Your Personal Journey with Food* readers as well as for clients of Tracy's or Ingrid's.)

Once you click on this link, select "Lab Testing" then "Individual Test Menu." Once you are on the Individual Test Menu page, scroll down to "Food Tolerance Testing," click on the plus sign.

Here you will see:

Adult Food Allergy Profile IgE
Advanced Food Sensitivity IgG—90+ foods plus Candida
Premium Food Sensitivity IgG—10 foods plus Candida

Select which test you would like to have, and Your Labwork will take care of everything for you.

I utilize both the elimination diet as well as blood tests with my clients. I have found that having a food sensitivity test to back up your theories is very helpful.

Also, having a doctor that specializes in food sensitivities as part of your team is VERY important! Food sensitivities can cause inflammation in the body, which can lead to chronic illness. Immediately look at all the foods you are eating if you have been diagnosed with a chronic disease.

You will also want to look for any other possible antagonists, as I mentioned earlier, such as pollutants, mold, toxic chemicals, etc. Irritants other than food can also cause symptoms. Things such as exposure to chemicals, prescription drugs, insect bites, and pet dander can all cause reactions.

I would like to tell you about two extreme reactions to chemicals that I had. I hope that my story will help you understand how symptoms can occur and help you or a loved one uncover possible chemical sensitivities.

#1 Citronella: We had always used citronella fuel in our patio torches. I had never noticed a problem with the torches until we moved to our little place on the water. We now have a small deck versus a large, open patio. One day, we had the torches lit on the deck for aesthetics. The door to the deck was open, and the wind was blowing from east to west, thus blowing the citronella fumes right into our living room. Without realizing this, as I was watching TV, I started to feel like I was coming down with a cold. My sinuses were burning, my throat was scratchy, and I was getting fatigued, nauseous, and cold. I decided to get a blanket and pillow and laid down on the couch. I fell asleep. About 30 minutes or so later, I woke up with a start. I felt terrible! I could taste the citronella in my mouth and realized what was happening. The Citronella had fumigated our entire apartment. My husband didn't notice a thing as he is not sensitive to it at all. In a panic, I went outside and put out the torches. I ended up having to sit in the far corner of the deck, while we opened all the windows in our place to air it out. Once aired out, I went to bed, still feeling terrible. When I woke up the next morning, I felt much better!

#2 Formaldehyde in New Carpet: A past employer of mine moved offices. When they moved to the new office, it was freshly painted, and new carpet and rubber baseboards were installed. As my first day in the new space progressed, I started to feel like I was getting a cold; my sinuses, throat, and eyes began to burn. Soon I had a headache and just wanted to go home and go to bed. I went home and did just that, thinking I had caught a flu bug or a cold.

When I woke up the next morning, I was fine. Thank goodness! I went back to the office that morning and was hit with a horrible taste, and the strong scent of chemicals, as I walked through the door. I tried to work, but as the hours progressed, I was soon sick again. I decided to go in the next day anyway, but the same thing happened. It took over a year for me to be able to work in that office space. I had to work remotely, as the carpet finished "off-gassing." We tested the air and found that the office did have an elevated level of Formaldehyde. Interestingly enough, it didn't bother any of the other staff members.

In both these examples, I had a horrible sense of impending doom. My instincts were to run, and I felt horribly claustrophobic. I must tell you I am not a claustrophobic person, and this was out of character for me.

This chapter started as information specific to food, but as you can see, it is wise to look at your external environment for possible chemical and environmental triggers that may be causing symptoms. Make sure you are not being exposed to unidentified antagonists. There is no need to spend a lifetime suffering. Educating yourself on how your own body responds to food is one of the most rewarding journeys. I didn't say it was easy, but it is worthwhile. Over time, your body can reset itself and start to function as it should. Give it the gift of this opportunity.

Exercise: Food Sensitivity Discovery

- ⊕ Commit to yourself that you will find out whether you have a food sensitivity or not.
- ⊕ Pick a date that you will either start an elimination diet or have your blood drawn so that you can get your food sensitivity panel done.
- ⊕ Pat yourself on the back! You are on your way to learning a great deal about your body! This is an exciting time!

Your Personal Journal With Food

Week Number:_____ Date:_____

What did you eat this week?

_____

_____

_____

How many glasses of plain water per day?_____
What did you do this week that makes you happy?

_____

_____

Percentage of processed foods this week:_____

Percentage of Mindful meals this week:_____

Elimination path:

1. Remove the following foods for three weeks: eggs, dairy, gluten, nuts, yeast, soy, corn, shellfish.
2. Add probiotics in capsule form
3. After three weeks begin introducing ONE food at a time. Introduce a new food each week. Use the following table to track how your body reacts to that food.

Food Reintroduction Chart

	Day 1 Food Added	Day 2 Symptoms	Day 3 Symptoms	Day 4 Symptoms	Add Back?
Week 1					
Week 2					
Week 3					
Week 4					

CHAPTER 8

Rest Stop—Get Up and Move
By Tracy

"Exercise is a CELEBRATION of what your body can do!
Not a punishment for what you ate."

I saw the above quote on the chalkboard at the gym several years ago. I don't know who said it, but I wish I did. This quote hit home for me. It made me think about my journey not only with exercise but with food and self-image. After reading it, I recalled all those moments when I exercised to punish myself, not only for what I ate but also for who I "was" and for who I "wasn't." Each exercise session was a brutal battle I waged against my body and my being as a whole.

But building over the past few years, I have grown to see exercise as a celebration of what my body CAN do. Exercise is a celebration of what my body does for me every second of every day. Exercising is celebrating the fact that my body allows me to travel on this incredible journey called Life and feeling tremendous gratitude for that. With that all said, I would like to share my modified version of the above quote. "Exercise is a CELEBRATION of what your body can do and NOT a punishment for what you ate. NOT a punishment for who you are. NOT a punishment for who you aren't."

Vehicles such as automobiles, bicycles, scooters, motorcycles, airplanes—you name it are meant to move. Your body is also meant to move. It is a priceless vehicle made to move! It is a miracle machine that takes you through your days as best it can by utilizing the fuel and direction you give it. Therefore, I ask, what direction do you give it? What fuel do you give it? What performance level do you expect from your body? Does your fuel line up with your expectations? Do you know if it does?

Just as our body and brain require high-quality nutrition to perform at their best, they need movement as well. We are not meant to be stationary, immobile beings. We are intended to be moving! Yes, I have said this several times already, but it is crucial to understand. Your overall health depends on it.

Many of our aches and pains come from the sedentary lifestyles we have developed. Our muscles waste away due to lack of movement. Our joints and tendons become tight. The dysfunction caused by sedentary behavior makes it difficult for our brain to communicate properly to all areas of the body. If we do not keep the body and brain communicating through movement, we lose our ability to do many things. When we move, we think better, learn better, and remember better.

The Lymphatic System

Movement is also imperative for a healthy immune system and a properly functioning lymphatic system.

Without movement, our bodies cannot process waste as efficiently. As Ingrid discusses in **Chapter 9, Tune-Up—Time to Detox**, we need to allow our bodies the opportunity to flush waste and toxins from the cells and thus from the body. However, it cannot function optimally without movement. When we sit or lay around all day, we continue to build up toxins, thus causing the challenges which Ingrid speaks of. When the lymphatic system is not functioning properly, it will inadvertently be contributing to weight gain as it won't be processing fat properly.

The lymphatic system does not have its' own pump. We must move our bodies to help it pump the fluid within it. Breathing, as well as the contraction of our muscles, make it function. Going for a walk, stretching, squeezing your muscles, bouncing on a small trampoline or jumping for just a few minutes a day will help it do its job. The system is incredible, and I HIGHLY recommend you do some of your own research and learn as much as you can about it. Because the lymphatic system is so vital to your overall health, the more you know, the more you will be able to make healthy decisions for your body.

Skeletal Muscles, Tendons, and the Brain-Body Connection

Without movement, we lose muscle tone, our tendons become tight, and we become more susceptible to injury. It is essential to exercise the communication between the brain and the rest of the body. Have you ever noticed that when you first try something new physically, it feels awkward and a bit unsettling? Notice that with repetition, your movement begins to improve. Your muscles start to understand what is expected of them as the brain is also better able to communicate its' intent. The reaction time from initial thought to actual movement becomes more natural, more subconscious vs. conscious.

Let's experiment; get up and stand next to the wall or where you can grab hold of a chair or other stable item if necessary. Now, lift one foot off the ground and raise your knee as if you are going to march. Try your best to hold this position as you lift one hand above your head. Do you feel stable or a bit off balance? Did you have to place your foot down? Did you sway a little and need to grab hold of something to stabilize? If so, that's OK!

Now, try again, but this time be present and a bit systematic. Feel your feet on the ground. Notice your toes and wiggle them. Notice the pressure of your weight on your feet. Is it centered, or do you put weight on the outside of your feet, for example? Disperse your weight evenly from the heel through the toes. Now, tell the leg that is going to be holding you up while the other raises its knee, that it has to keep you steady. Start to activate your muscles in that leg in preparation. Squeeze your calf muscles, thighs, hamstrings, and glutes (buttock muscles) in your support leg. Now tighten your core (abdominal muscles) and tell them that they are going to help stabilize you as well. NOW, begin to raise the other foot up and off the ground. Keep your focus on the supporting leg. This is the leg that will help you keep your balance. Not the one you are lifting. Stay firm and tight through that leg. Keep your mind focused on the foot and floor. Notice that you may have improved slightly. Try again and pay attention to the muscles in your stabilizing leg. What is happening to them? Notice how they flex. How about your ankle? Is it adjusting to keep you balanced? Does it even know what it needs to do to perform the task you are asking of it? Do you notice anything else? What about your core muscles? Your glutes? (buttock muscles).

Keep trying this exercise, switching between both legs. Is one leg more stable than the other? Practice over and over until you can easily lift your knee and raise one of your arms over your head and hold for at least 30 seconds, then switch arms, switch legs. Pretty soon, the communication between your brain and the necessary muscles improves. The communication becomes quicker and more reliable each time, and you will become more stable as the effort to do so becomes less and less.

With all this said, it is essential to remember that movement of the body is not only good for burning calories, strengthening muscles, stabilizing joints, and for losing weight, but it is also good for the brain. The exercise you just did shows this. We have to use the brain and make sure it knows how to communicate with all the moving parts of our bodies. If you have a tough time performing this exercise, and you do not see any improvement after many attempts, you should find a professional to help you figure out what is causing the miscommunication.

Movement and Food

Because food integrates with every part of the body, your nutrition is directly related to your ability and desire to exercise. Have you heard how athletes will plan their meals around their training requirements and competitions? They will look ahead and eat according to what their physical demands will be.

For example, when I began to do endurance cycling rides of up to 100 miles, I knew I had to have fuel for my body to make it through the physical demands of the ride. I would plan for this. Several days before the 100-mile ride, I would begin to eat the foods necessary so that on the day of the ride, I could perform as planned. During times when I was not riding, I ate differently. I didn't need the same types of calories on a daily basis, as I did when I was putting in the time on the bike.

I have also found that if I eat food that I am sensitive to, such as dairy or eggs, I will feel sluggish and sick to my stomach. I won't have the energy or desire to exercise. In the past, when I ate these foods, my mind was sometimes able to win over my body, and I forced myself to exercise. These workouts were difficult, drawn-out battles of mind over matter. It took all I had to make it through. If I ate clean, mainly whole foods, and not from my sensitivity list, I found that I had a lot more energy, and my body performed better. Eating this way would make my workouts much more fun and rewarding.

Getting Started

How is your fitness regimen? Do you have a hard time staying consistent? Do you have a hard time just getting started?

Sometimes it's hard to start a regimen because we believe we have to go to the gym for an hour or more each time. The fact is that you do not need a gym membership to start exercising. All you need is you! That's it! Isn't that exciting?! Later in this chapter, I will give you the opportunity to download the complimentary booklet, **All You Need is You!** which includes exercises you can do right at home, or at your office, at the park, pretty-much anywhere without any equipment at all! These exercises can also be done in a small hallway or entry. You don't need a lot of room.

There are also great on-demand, YouTube, and downloadable workout programs you can do right from your home. These include yoga, spinning, dancing, Zumba, martial arts, you name it! What is it you like to do? Is there a way you can create an environment at home if getting to the gym is not something you can or want to do?

Movement Dysfunction

Kinetic Chain Dysfunction. What in the world is that? Our bodies are meant to move in certain ways. If something is going on with the body that causes it to move outside of its natural way, that is called Kinetic Chain Dysfunction. Most everyone has some form of Kinetic Chain Dysfunction. In my case, I have had to relearn to walk normally several times. I have had injuries in both knees, Achilles tendonitis in both tendons at the same time, sciatica challenges, and a big toe joint issue. All of these injuries caused me to compensate when I walked. Over time, I just walked funny, which would cause me to pull the muscles in my ankles consistently. Once I finally realized I needed some help, went to sports therapy, I learned to walk the right way again.

When injuries are involved, the mind will quickly start to utilize other areas of the body to compensate for the injured area. When doing this, muscles and tendons that are not meant to perform certain movements are asked to do so, thus causing stress injuries to them. It can be a spiral of on-going chronic movement injuries.

Injuries are not the only thing that causes kinetic chain dysfunction. Let's look at it from the sedentary lifestyle aspect. Sitting, for example, shortens the thigh muscles and the core muscles. It lengthens the lower back muscles, and it compresses the lower spine by forcing the back into a curvature that it was not meant to be in for long hours of the day. At a desk, we often have to hold our heads up at a forward and downward angle. This position causes strain to the neck muscles, which creates tension down into the upper shoulders and between the shoulders. In the meantime, the chest muscles (which are naturally stronger than the back and shoulder muscles) tighten and start to pull your shoulders forward, causing more stress on the upper and mid-shoulder muscles. Everything starts to hurt. Pretty soon, sleep is difficult. Walking becomes difficult. Lifting becomes difficult—all of this just from sitting for long hours every day.

Exercise: Journaling

You will want to get out your journal for this. If you don't have a journal to use, download your free **"Your Personal Journey with Food Journal"** from **www.journeywithfood.com**.

- List ALL the reasons you can think of that are stopping you from exercising or preventing you from progressing to a higher fitness level. Do not be critical of yourself; don't silence your thoughts or leave anything off the list. If something comes to mind, write it down, no matter how small. (example: no time, afraid to go to the gym, don't know what to do, don't feel right, lazy, finances, scared, don't feel good enough, etc.)

- Which of the reasons on your list weighs the heaviest on you emotionally, and which the least? Go ahead and rate them highest to lowest and relist them in that order. Do you see any particular trends?

- Now, of the reasons listed, are there any based-on fear? Write the word "Fear" next to these.

- Are there any that you need help with and believe you would move past if you just had some additional knowledge or assistance from someone? Write "Assistance" next to these.

- Do any of these reasons come from a place of hopelessness? Do you believe that there is absolutely no way to move past these reasons? If so, write "Hopeless" next to these.

- Are there any reasons which you realize aren't such a big deal now that you see them on paper? You just didn't know you were allowing them to get in the way. Write, "I got this!" next to these.

- Now, next to all of your reasons on the list, write, "I can conquer, I just need to learn how."

- Some reasons will have more than one word next to them. The purpose of this exercise is to isolate what is driving your decision not to allow or prioritize body movement. As with any challenge you are facing, you have to know what is driving your choices.

As you review your list, what pattern of reasons do you see? Count how many times a word is utilized and list them in order.

What are your thoughts about the results? Consider the following:

Fear: Does your fear have merit? Are you really going to die or be injured if you move forward through these reasons to a more active lifestyle? Write either yes or no next to each reason based on fear. If no, what can you do to break through the fear? Can you get assistance? Can you do some research on what is blocking you and find a solution? If you honestly believe yes, that you will be injured, then most definitely look for professional assistance and see if there is a way to get your body moving without fear of fatality or injury.

Assistance: What type of assistance do you need? A friend or loved one's support? How about hiring a professional to help you overcome pain or a hopeless feeling of fatigue or lethargy? What do you need? Write this down. Now, within the next 24 hours, reach out to who you think can help and start the conversation. Don't wait.

Hopeless: Write down why you believe it's hopeless to try to move past each reason. Allow your mind to search for solutions to each of these. Is it hopeless? Can these items be removed from your list if you had some assistance?

I Got This: Fantastic! What is your plan of action to make this change? Write it down and commit. Start right now. If you need a few days to set things in motion and make the change, fine—but commit.

You now have a good picture of what your mindset is regarding your physical activity level. You also have the beginning of a plan to get you started on your movement journey. You are continuing to learn about yourself, your body, and how your mind functions! A significant, as well as a positive step forward, has been made, so let's celebrate! We tend not to give ourselves enough credit for these types of accomplishments.

Now, it's time to get started. Figure out your plan and move those roadblocks out of the way. Address each reason as you determined was necessary. Rally your support team, call a professional, etc. You may have to start small, and that's OK. Every little step forward counts. No one can climb a mountain with just one big step. It takes many smaller steps over time and behind the scenes training and coaching. Absolutely!

Ways to Get Moving

I have put together a complimentary booklet full of exercises to help you get started. The exercises I am recommending require no additional equipment. Just you! You don't need to go to the gym, and you don't need to spend a lot of money on expensive equipment. Isn't that great?! Not getting to the gym doesn't have to be an obstacle for you anymore. Invest the money you would waste on an un-used gym membership on healthy, whole foods instead. You cannot exercise yourself out of a bad diet. (Believe me, many have tried and failed, me included!)

To get your "**Movement! All I Need is Me!**" booklet, visit **www. journeywithfood.com.**

Reminders

I have reminders set up on my smartphone. Life is busy, and an hour can fly by before I know it and then even two. Within those hours, I may be working at my desk and forget to move. I set reminders to get up and walk as well as for various exercises dependent on my environment at the time. What reminders can you set for yourself to help you remember to move?

Now, go back to your journal exercise and write, "I will conquer! I just need to learn how! I just need to get started! It's just taking small steps, and I can do that! I can take small, consistent steps!"

Oh! And don't forget to download your free booklet, **Movement! All I Need is Me!**

Your Personal Journal With Food

Week Number:_____ Date:_____

What did you eat this week?

_____

_____

_____

_____

_____

How many glasses of plain water per day?_____
What did you do this week that makes you happy?

_____

_____

Percentage of processed foods this week:_____

Percentage of Mindful meals this week:_____

Better Performance Tracker

	Mon	Tue	Wed	Thu	Fri	Sat	Sun
Physical Activity							

CHAPTER 9

Tune-Up—Time to Detox
By Ingrid and Tracy

Let's make a road stop in our journey and DETOX.

The word "detox" has become a buzz word within the diet and wellness industry. There seem to be hundreds of available detox programs (and opinions) on the market. With all these options and opinions, how do you know if a detox is right for you, let alone which one?

First, let's establish what a "detox" is. I found this definition of the word in the Merriam-Webster Dictionary:[1]

> 1A: *to remove a harmful substance (as a poison or toxin) or the effect of such from b: to render (a harmful substance) harmless*
> *2: to free (as a drug user or an alcoholic) from an intoxicating or an addictive substance in the body or from dependence on or addiction to such a substance*
> *3: Neutralize*

---

1. https://www.merriam-webster.com/dictionary/detox

Regarding *Your Personal Journey with Food*, we will:

a. Look at what a detox is and why we consider it essential to add to your lifestyle.

b. We will outline several types of detox programs

c. At the end of the chapter, we will suggest a holistic and safe method of detox to include in your own *Personal Journey with Food*.

Why Detox?

We live in a world of alternating cycles of light and darkness. The day and night are natural markers for our schedules of activity and rest. Due to our ability to create artificial light, we can modify this cycle, allowing us to be active at night. However, at some point, we will feel the need to rest and sleep. Through experience, we are aware that sleeping in the daytime is not as restful as sleeping during the night. Those who work a night shift know this firsthand. Even if they are used to their schedule, at some point, this lifestyle will have adverse effects on their health.

Seasons of the year also determine the cycles of our activity and rest. Our body cells can sense these changes and act differently according to the weather. Scientists[2] have observed that the immune system has more pro-inflammatory proteins (cells that are more alert and armed, ready to defend the body) during and after rainy seasons, as well as in the cold temperatures of winter. After all, we are a part of nature, and our body performs at its best when we are in balance with it, recognizing and respecting nature's cycles and living in harmony with each one.

The Chinese philosophy of Yin-Yang explains how two opposing energies can be in balance. One negative, dark, and feminine (yin) and one positive, bright, and masculine (yang), and whose interaction influences the destinies of creatures and things. As long as there is Yang, an active period, there should be Yin, a rest period. I'm not only talking about how

---

2. Dopico, reveals the differences in human immunity and physiology based on seasons. X. C. et al. Widespread seasonal gene expression Nat. Commun. 6:7000 doi: 10.1038/ncomms8000 (2015)

vital sleeping is to have good energy and health, but also referring to the Yin-Yang function of our digestive system. In our hectic and unhealthy culture, our digestive systems get little or no rest.

So how does all of this relate to our digestive system and detoxing? In Westernized societies, (the world in which we live), there is an overabundance of many things, including food. The digestive system can take anywhere from 4 to 6 hours to process a meal. The meal is usually a combination of the three macronutrients: protein, carbohydrates, and fats. It can take even longer for these foods to digest, depending on the amount and type of fats (up to 9 hours). With this in mind, think about your typical day and how many hours your body may spend digesting.

Below is a classic example of a typical day in the life of a human digestive system in South America:

8:00 am—Breakfast (digestive process ends between 12 pm and 2 pm)

11:00 am—Snack (digestive process ends between 1 pm and 3 pm)

1:30 pm—Lunch (digestive process ends between 6:30 pm and 7:30 pm)

5:00 pm—At this time, we have a meal similar to breakfast. We call it "Merienda" or "Once," (digestive process ends between 8 pm and 10 pm)

9:00 pm—Dinner (digestive process ends between 2 am and 4 am)

In this example, a digestive system works between 18 to 22 hours per day and only rests 2 to 4 hours between meals. However, this is only if a person does not eat anything after 11 pm. If they do have that 11 pm snack, they will be digesting food the entire 24 hours of their day!

Why This Information is so Valuable

The process of digestion uses a significant amount of energy to obtain nutrients from the food you eat. When digestion takes place, it is the number one priority of the body. Other metabolic processes, such as removing toxins, a natural capability of our bodies, are put on hold until digestion ends.

If 8 hours of sleep is recommended to maintain good health, maybe we should let our digestive system rest for 8 hours as well? Meaning, we should have our last meal between 6 and 7 pm. No midnight snacks!

When we do this, we synchronize with our circadian clock. Chinese medicine states that the energetic channels of different organs are more active during certain periods of the day and night. In the picture below, we see that some organs participating in the depuration process are more active at nighttime. When we are resting, bile release occurs. Bile aids in digestion and fat assimilation and is an elimination vehicle for liver waste and cholesterol. Note that liver and lung detoxification take place while in a deep sleep. These two organs are essential for the removal of toxins out of our bodies. If the digestive process occupies these two organs, the body will not detoxify properly.

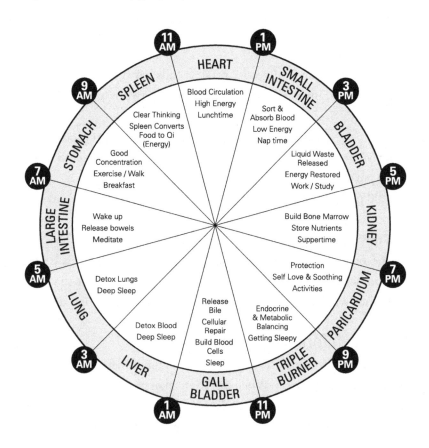

Perhaps after a large, heavy dinner, you have experienced difficulty in getting restful sleep. You wake in the morning with poor energy. Your low energy is due not only to poor sleep. The toxins that remain in your system, which could not be removed during the night, are also a reason for your lack of energy.

Why Do I Have Toxins in My Body?

Toxins are the body's normal byproducts that are not nutritious and can even be harmful. Toxins also come from our environment as well as from the food we choose to eat.

With that in mind, let´s review some of the toxins that form inside the body. When we eat food and digest it, our body produces toxins. These toxins are called metabolic toxins and are byproducts of every metabolic pathway in the mind and body. Food isn't the only source of these toxins. Stress and repressed emotions like anger, sadness, and guilt can become the toxic waste of the mind.

Certain digestive functions like fatty acid metabolism, amino acid metabolism, and carbohydrate metabolism (among others) create toxins. In addition, toxin levels can be increased and compounded if we have nutritional imbalances or inherited enzyme deficits. Ingesting such things as toxic elements, chemical toxicants, medications, or any substance that disrupts the biochemical balance like sugar, refined flour, or chemical additives like flavorings, colorings, preservatives, etc., also increases toxin levels in the body.

Not only are we exposed to toxins internally from our food, but external toxins from the environment also challenge our bodies. We live in a contaminated world. A world in which many of our cities have air loaded with smog, water that is contaminated with heavy metals, and homes filled with textiles that emit VOCs (Volatile Organic Compounds). Many household cleaning products and cosmetics are highly toxic and are absorbed quickly through our skin.

Thankfully, our bodies have internal organs specifically designed to remove these toxins. But all of these toxins in our surroundings make these organs work very hard. Add a not so healthy diet like the SAD

(Standard American Diet) and the SCD (Standard Chilean Diet), plus the fact we are eating all day long results in toxic load within our bodies.

The smartest thing we can do is learn how to recognize and deal with toxins in our environment and food. We can help our bodies by doing a detox once in a while. Detoxing is a tool that can help us stay healthy in the world in which we currently live.

Signs of Body Toxicity

- Feeling tired even with enough sleep
- Cravings
- Feeling hungry all the time
- Strong body odor
- Headaches
- Frequent colds, infections or viruses
- Constipation
- Allergies or hay fever
- Congestion
- Feeling bloated after eating
- Those few extra pounds you can't lose with diet and exercise
- Puffiness
- Itchy skin
- Pain or stiffness in your joints or muscles
- Restless sleep
- Lows moods or a foggy mind
- Difficulty concentrating
- Feeling excessively tired and apathetic
- Moodiness and bursts of irrational anger and frustration

What if Toxicity Remains in Our Bodies?

According to the Natural Hygiene Movement Theory, the accumulation of toxins affects our body to the extent that we develop diseases. Within the theory, they identify seven stages of disease:

Stage 1—Enervation
Tiredness or exhaustion. An extreme state of enervation is "nervous exhaustion." Sleep regenerates nerve energy. Lack of sleep, ongoing stress, and an unhealthy lifestyle all contribute to enervation.

Stage 2—Toxemia or toxicosis
The body produces a lot of toxic byproducts, such as carbon dioxide. Toxic waste builds up in the body due to an unhealthy lifestyle.

Stage 3—Irritation
Irritation results from un-eliminated waste products being sensed by our central nervous system. When we feel unsettled, itchy, queasy, jumpy, or uncomfortable without being able to detect the source, irritation exists. Excess mucus or an itchy nose is a form of irritation. Substances like alcohol, caffeine, or cigarettes can trigger irritation of the body.

Stage 4—Inflammation
This stage is recognizable usually by pain and or redness and swelling. Any condition ending in "itis" such as sinusitis, tonsillitis, appendicitis is a form of inflammation. Running a temperature would fall into this stage.

Stage 5—Ulceration
This stage develops if stage 4 is not dealt with and usually means mass destruction of cells. Lesions or ulcers can occur anywhere in the body. This condition often results in pain.

Stage 6—Induration
Induration is when the body tries to patch itself up. The scarring and hardening of tissue are the result. Very often, the body will wrap cells around toxic substances, which then harden, forming a tumor.

Stage 7—Mutation
In this stage, to survive the acidic and poorly oxygenated environment, the cells start to behave independently and multiply. They mutate, and this is the time when degenerative diseases like cancer develop.

Although this theory is not scientifically confirmed, it links disease with the overload of toxins in the body through poor food choices and bad eating habits. It is interesting to me that many allopathic doctors (and several studies) now say that many common lifestyle diseases (which you've probably heard of), are directly related to bad eating habits and junk food.

Listed below are some of the most common lifestyle diseases:

- Atherosclerosis
- Alzheimer's disease
- Some types of cancer
- Asthma
- Liver cirrhosis
- Type 2 diabetes
- Chronic obstructive pulmonary disease
- Heart disease
- Metabolic syndrome
- Chronic renal failure
- Stroke
- Osteoporosis
- Obesity
- Depression

What is good news for us? We have just two things to do that will benefit our health: begin eating a balanced diet and living a healthy lifestyle.

And the key to reducing toxicity? Nurture yourself with a clean diet, and do not overeat. A clean diet means eating organic produce as much as possible, cooking meals from whole foods at home, eating lots of vegetables, removing processed sugars and flours from your diet, and no alcohol or smoking.

Tracy and I understand that eating clean daily is challenging and can be hard to do at first, but it is worth it. You can be an inspiration to your circle of beloved people and help them to improve their habits and lifestyles, too.

Keep in mind that avoiding toxins in food will only decrease the number of toxins entering through your mouth. There will still be external toxins entering your body through your lungs, skin, and mind. That is why I recommend doing a detox once a year and doing your best to practice a 70% clean diet.

Detox Methods

There are a lot of detox methods. I have tried several of the following myself.

Homemade Plant-Based Diet

Pros: This diet is sustainable for lengthy periods. It significantly reduces the number of processed foods consumed. Vegetables and fruit are 70 to 80 percent of your food intake and thus make it the perfect choice for a core diet.[3]

Cons: This diet takes time to plan and prepare, but it's worth it! Also, according to some researchers and doctors, people with certain health conditions such as thyroid-related and autoimmune diseases need to eat some animal products. If they don't, they may have trouble digesting some vegetables and fruits due to food sensitivities, allergies, or leaky gut syndrome. So, this may not be for everyone.

If food is not homemade or includes too many nuts, sugar, and flour, you could end up being what is called a junk-food vegan. A junk-food vegan is a person that eats a lot of processed vegan food vs. real whole foods. Eating this way also creates chronic inflammation in the body.

By eating homemade vegan food, you reduce a lot of toxic sources (such as processed food and animal protein) from your diet. (Processed

---

3. There is a lot of information on this subject. If you want to know more about this, do an Internet search with the keywords Gluten and Thyroid.

and animal protein sources are difficult for your digestive system to metabolize.) Eating homemade vegan food will also help to reduce and even eliminate most preservatives, artificial flavorings, artificial colorings, and chemicals that are usually added to processed foods.

You can start transitioning to eating a vegan diet by eliminating meat and trying a vegetarian diet first. Temporarily removing animal protein from your diet eases the workload on your digestive system. Remember that animal protein is hard for most people to digest, and in the process of digesting these proteins, toxins are produced. Another benefit of removing meat temporarily from your diet is so that you can find out if your body needs some animal proteins. If so, you will be able to figure out which kind might be beneficial to your health. By eliminating meat in this way, I discovered that fish benefits my digestion. Tracy found that whey protein, which, according to science, is the easiest to digest protein, does not work for her body at all and gives her diarrhea and stomach cramps.

Fruits and vegetable nutrients tend to assimilate better into the human body; they help to balance the ph of the blood as well as reduce and prevent chronic inflammation. A study of the vegan diet[4] shows that in only three months, this meal plan helps to reverse prostate cancer, and 90% of patients who needed a critical operation did not need it after eating a vegan diet.

A series of published, randomized controlled trials in leading peer-reviewed journals has scientifically proven that a plant-based diet reverses the progression of severe coronary heart disease, type 2 diabetes, hypercholesterolemia, and high blood pressure. Science has also found that changing your lifestyle also changes your genetic expression. Meaning that you are turning on protective genes and turning off those that promote inflammation, oxidative stress, and oncogenes that promote prostate cancer, breast cancer, and colon cancer—over 500 genes in only three months. In addition, these lifestyle changes lengthen telomeres on our chromosomes that regulate aging, thereby helping to reverse aging at a cellular level.

---

4. Ornish Vegan Diet, according to www.ornishlifestyle.com

How to Apply It

I recommend you add plant-based foods slowly. In your first attempt, 50% of your plate should be plant-based foods and then increase gradually.

Nutrients coming from raw fruits and raw vegetables have better absorption by the human body due to their naturally packed enzymes. However, in people with weak or damaged digestive systems, leaky gut syndrome, lack of enzymes, or poor gut flora or food sensitivities, eating raw foods could lead to gas, bloating, or even interfere in nutrient absorption. For that reason, some people will need to consume cooked vegetables. Those with thyroid dysfunction should consume cooked vegetables from the cruciferous family: kale, broccoli, cauliflower, cabbage.

If you have a food sensitivity or food allergy caused by a specific fruit or vegetable, be sure to remove that vegetable or fruit from your diet. If you don't remove it, it will increase your toxic load. There are several ways to identify food sensitivities and allergies. **Chapter 7, Picking the Right Fuel—Food Sensitivities.**

To receive the highest benefit from this way of eating, choose fresh organic produce. You don't have to buy everything organic, just those fruits and vegetables that have a thin layer of skin. Tomatoes, berries, or spinach (among others) will absorb a higher amount of pesticides than those with thicker skins. For a complete list, please visit the Environmental Working Group website.[5]

Take the time to plan your meals so that they have variety and nutritional balance. Experimenting with recipes will add fun and creativity.

Is it wise to make a vegan diet permanent? There are opposing arguments. People changing from the SAD or SCD diet usually report improvements in health conditions associated with chronic inflammation like type 2 diabetes and other conditions. For others, there is evidence that being vegan is not sustainable over a lifetime. Every person is a private universe concerning their food and health, so we suggest trying it mindfully for 3 to 6 months. If you currently consume a high amount

---

5. www.ewg.org.

of processed food, the benefits of only one month on this vegan program will be life-changing.

Juicing

Juicing is very trendy these days. You spend a few days utilizing liquid nutrition from fruits and vegetable juices only. When juicing, I prefer cold-pressed to preserve more nutrients. Juicing separates the fiber from the fruit or vegetable, along with the nutrients and the natural sugar (fructose). In fruit, the natural fiber helps our body absorb the sugar and nutrients gradually. Because of this, it is not recommended to drink a cold-pressed juice made only of fruits. If you do, you will be drinking too much sugar, and this can create high and low insulin peaks in your blood. These peaks will then cause dramatic high and low energy levels.

The benefit of drinking juice is that you will not spend much energy on digestion. Your digestive system will get a break, and the nutrients from the juice will absorb into your bloodstream within a short amount of time.

A juice detox is perfect for those who suffer from malnutrition or lack of vitamins and minerals. Juicing also helps you get large quantities of vegetables into your system. Consuming greens this way is easier, and you can double the daily portion of vegetables by drinking them, rather than eating them. A large juice can have half a plant of celery, three to five carrots, several handfuls of leafy veggies like kale or spinach, one cucumber, and two apples. A lot of nutrition in just one serving!!!

You can purchase juices made by specific manufacturers. They usually offer 3 to 5-day programs. If you have a juicer at home, you can make it yourself. Just be sure to use at least 50 to 60-percent vegetables in the ingredients. Otherwise, sugar in the fruit can create an insulin imbalance because of the excess of sugar in your blood.

Drink enough juice to satisfy your hunger. You may need to drink more because you are having liquid nutrition and no fiber. For me, a satisfying amount of juice is 5 to 6 liters (1.3 to 1.5 gallons) per day. I also enjoy having one to two glasses of nut or seed milk (such as hemp milk) to make sure I am getting enough protein.

You may try this detox for 3 to 7 days.

Cons: Poor amounts of fiber, proteins, and healthy fats. Depending on the ingredients of juice, the amount of sugars could be high. This detox is not sustainable for extended time periods.

Mono Diets

This kind of diet is popular in India as a way to enhance a spiritual experience. Only one food is consumed for 40 days, such as apple, or basmati rice or lentils. I do not have any experience with this kind of detox personally. Nor have I found scientific evidence confirming that eating the same food for a specific amount of time will detoxify the body. Nutritionally speaking, I believe that eating just one type of food for such a long time could bring nutritional imbalance to the body.

Flushes

Flushes are frequently used with some detox protocols to increase bowel function. The objective is to empty the gut and flush out feces and toxins quickly. This method is usually used with a megadose of vitamin C, or salted water, or just high volumes of water. If you are tempted to try a flush, please research it beforehand and evaluate the pros and cons. There is the risk of dehydration, demineralization, and loss of precious gut flora.

Liver Detox Protocol

As I said earlier in this chapter, the liver is one of the primary organs involved in detoxifying the body. For that reason, there is a detox protocol specifically focused on removing toxins from it. The protocol involves ingesting Epsom salts (and other ingredients) that act as a laxative and allows for the removal of toxins.

It is best to prepare yourself for this cleanse with a vegan diet for one week and one or two sessions of colonics. Then for five days, you will drink green apple juice in the morning until noon, followed by a 90% raw vegan lunch, snack, and dinner. After that, you will spend half a day fasting and should drink a mixture of grapefruit juice with olive oil followed by Epsom salts diluted in water. The protocol is very specific regarding quantities and timing. It is essential to follow those rules precisely.

After you drink the Epsom salts, you have to lie down on your right side and get some rest. Soon you will feel the need to go to the bathroom and may release what are called "stones." Some people have taken these green and brown stones to a laboratory for analysis, and results show they consist mainly of triglycerides. Triglycerides are the main ingredient of a naturally occurring fat in humans and animals.

The protocol ends the following day at noon, at which time you may eat something light and vegan again. But 24 to 36 hours after that, it is crucial to do another colonic session to clean your bowel and prevent reabsorption of remaining stones and toxins.

For me, the most valuable outcome from doing this cleanse was that it helped me to address an old pain in the kidney area that no doctor could diagnose. Many times, I had to go to the hospital because of this pain. The symptoms were the same as if I had stones in my gallbladder. The pain was such that all I wanted to do was run away from my body.

I did this protocol with the guidance of a professional colonics expert. To learn more about the complete protocol, research the liver detox protocol of Andreas Moritz or read the work of Dr. Hulda Clark.

This protocol has worked for me, but I can't speak for you. I am sharing my experience with you for informational purposes only. If you decide to do this cleanse, I highly recommend finding a professional to assist you. Do not attempt to do it on your own.

Panchakarma

Panchakarma is a method of cleansing from Ayurvedic (also called Ayurveda) medicine, which is an ancient, holistic (whole-body) healing wisdom for wellness and longevity originating in India. Panchakarma (five actions) is a cleansing and rejuvenating program for the body, mind, and consciousness. It helps remove what is called "Ama." Ama is the result of inadequate digestion resulting from heavy meals, poor food combinations, and/or a weak digestive system resulting in gas, bloating, constipation, and heartburn. Ama Ayurvedic medicine describes Ama as a harmful force that can accumulate in the body. It can be a source of illnesses such as candida, chronic headaches, respiratory issues, chronic fatigue syndrome, among others.

The five actions system of Panchakarma eliminates Ama and helps the body to be in balance. This holistic system includes a special diet, massages, herbal supplements, and steam baths for 7 to 30 days.

The goal is to move the Ama back to the digestive system. Once there, the Ama is flushed out of the body by using purgatives/laxatives and herbal colonics. This method is performed in Holistic Health Centers or Ayurveda Centers (mostly found in India) at which you remain in for the entire time the treatment lasts.

Fasting

When Tracy and I studied together at the Institute for Integrative Nutrition, we reviewed several diet protocols, some of which opposed each other. One notable example is the two diet protocols, referred to as Paleo and Naturalism.

The Paleo diet (sometimes referred to as the "Stone Age Diet") promotes a whole foods diet that includes only meat, vegetables, fruits, and seeds. These are foods that were supposedly the only ones available during the Paleolithic period of history, and the only foods that were available to our ancestors. The diet avoids grains, dairy, and legumes.

Naturalism also utilizes whole foods, but does not implement any meat and embraces grains, legumes and is open to many food combinations.

The interesting part is that both of these lifestyles promote fasting as a detox and health improvement habit.

Fasting as a ritual has been present in many diverse cultures of the world throughout history. Hippocrates (460 bc–370 bc) advocated fasting as a way to recover one's health. Many religions have used (and still use) fasting as a purification method. More recently, in Russia and Germany, Dr. Yuri Nikolayev and Dr. Otto Buchinger have had amazing results with fasting in the treatment of mental illnesses like schizophrenia, and inflammatory diseases such as arthritis and atherosclerosis. Their studies show that they were able to cure many cases just by prescribing water fasting. The improvement rate of Dr. Nikolayev's treatment was 80%; over half of the patients were cured. Sadly, the beliefs of some doctors and the pharmaceutical industry, these studies remain in their original languages, thus difficult to find.

Fasting also normalizes sugar and cholesterol markers and has been shown to benefit cancer patients undergoing chemotherapy. Valter Longo, Ph.D., from California University, found that the gene expression of healthy cells changes with fasting and protects them from chemotherapy, while the gene expression of carcinogenic cells does not, therefore making chemotherapy more effective.

Fasting challenges our Occidental mindset. But if you observe nature, you will see that many animals fast, especially when they are sick or giving birth. Maybe your body will ask you to fast if you overeat. Fasting is mainly about allowing your digestive system to rest as nature intended. Fasting allows the body to use its energy for detoxification and removal of waste. When you fast, a process called cellular autophagy occurs. Autophagy (from the Greek roots, auto: self and Phago: to eat), basically means your body starts a recycle process and eliminate old and defective cells, thus renewing itself.

In my opinion, fasting is a powerful tool for detoxifying the body and for expanding your mind. With that said, detoxifying must be taken very seriously. Those who are pregnant or breastfeeding, have metabolic syndrome, diabetes, insulin dependence, or anorexia or bulimia problems must not fast. Neither should those people who are taking medications such as antidepressants, anxiolytics, or sleeping pills.

Different Types of Fasting

Intermittent fasting: Intermittent fasting is where you eat only at specific times of the day. All other times of the day, you will be fasting. It may also have you abstaining from food for 24 hours. There have been many studies done showing the health benefits of intermittent fasting, benefitting the brain in particular. Intermittent fasting also promotes long-term fat metabolism and the development of muscle mass.

Liquid Fasting: Liquid fasting means that you will drink only plain water, juice, or herbal infusions for a certain number of days. During this time, your body will be nurtured only by its current reserves. During a liquid fast, you can utilize a juice fast or the Master Cleanse Program (water with some amount of maple syrup, lemon juice, and cayenne pepper). The Master Cleanse Program has a duration of 10 days drinking that mixture and desired amounts of water. I have tried this program for detox purposes and have similar results as the liver detox protocol, but the experience was gentler and more gradual.

This method (as well as fasting methods) are not "diets" and are not intended to be utilized for weight control. Their purpose is to allow your body to detox naturally.

Some health professionals do not consider juicing a fast because your body is still nurtured with fruits and vegetables. However, I believe that juicing is a fast because you are only ingesting the liquid of the fruits and vegetables and resting your digestive system.

Water fasting is the most challenging. According to the documentary, "Fasten und Heilen—Altes Wissen und neueste Forshung," (Fasting and Healing—Old knowledge and latest Research), by Thierry de Lestrade and Sylvie Gilman, a person with an average weight could perform a 40-day water fast and not only improve their health but not damage muscle mass. Lestrade and Gilman believe this to be true because the body would be consuming energy from body fat reserves. However, long-term fasting such as this requires medical supervision. Some fasting clinics in Europe provide these services. These clinics supplement your fast with vitamins, a vegetable broth, exercise, and plenty of rest as necessary for each patient.[6]

Of course, you could perform a shorter fast. With that said, keep in mind that it takes about three days for the body to use up its reserve of glucose and glycogen. At that time, it will start to create energy from body fat as well as detox deeply.

---

6. Buchinger-Wilhelmi Fasting Clinic in Germany is one of the oldest and most experienced in long term fasting.

Dry Fasting: Dry fasting is when you don't eat or drink anything for specific amounts of time. I have not tried this fast, and I believe it is extreme. I do know several people who have done it. I have my doubts about this method because liquids are not being consumed; therefore, there is no vehicle to flush out toxins.

At this time, Tracy would like to discuss our detox proposal.

Although this book is called Your Personal Journey with Food, many aspects of life are not technically food-related but have a dramatic impact on your food choices, your body, and your life as a whole.

Understanding that everything in my life is connected—my food, my relationships, my environment, my thoughts, my physical body, my spirituality, and my finances; I am better able to discern what's right for me and what is not. I can recognize toxicity around me and am therefore more able to remove those toxicities from my life.

My "detoxification" didn't happen overnight. It has been and will continue to be an ongoing process.

Looking at life with the eyes of a curious student and being willing to try new things is important. Release judgment of one's self and being open to failure, as well as being open to succeeding, will aid you on this journey. (Yes, sometimes we can be afraid of succeeding at something just because it means change.) The road to health means embracing change.

There are a few routes you can take to a detoxified life. The quick, all at once, straight up the mountain path. The moderate switchback road, or the gradual circle around the mountain until you get to the top. The pace is up to you and your specific circumstances. You can always change your route along your journey.

Sometimes it can be easy to go fast, but when we don't have the skills necessary to maintain a new lifestyle, failure may be the result. I am all about testing skills, so if you want to go for it and take the quick route, please do. The quick path will expose the areas in which you need to learn more. Be prepared to struggle to maintain your new, detoxified lifestyle. Also, be ready to fail. Yes, I said, fail. But when you stumble, it's OK! All I ask is that you take note and ask yourself what caused you to stumble. Seek out the knowledge that will help you overcome obstacles next time and then bring that knowledge forward and go for it again. I promise, eventually, you will figure it out.

Any route you decide to take will be an adventure! Make it a fun one, and enjoy learning about yourself along the way. As you take this journey, be sure to stay in touch with Mindfulness. Mindfulness will be your compass. If you have not read **Chapter 5, Time for an Alignment—The Path of Mindfulness** yet, please stop reading this chapter and do that now. When done, join me back here.

Exercise: Time to Detox

For each area below, you will set a goal to detoxify. Your Quick Route may be faster than someone else's quick route. Your slow route may be slower or faster than someone else's slow route. Everyone is different. Just decide to get started.

STRAIGHT UP—THE QUICK ROUTE—this would be an ascent of 30 days to 1 year.
OK, this route is going to be fast. However, it can be a bit of a shock; a shock to your habits, known lifestyle, and possibly your wallet. Not that these are bad things. This investment in you, a priceless being, should be a priority.

MODERATE—THE SWITCHBACK ROUTE—this may be a walk of 1 to 3 years
This route will give you a good workout and a challenge, but much more manageable for some.

A SLOW AND STEADY CLIMB—this may be a walk of 5 years or more.
(My path was filled with all of these routes. In some areas, I was

able to make quick changes easily. In others, I was only able to move at a moderate to slow pace. Falling and regressing many times, then regrouping and going for it again.)

The Body

Foods—85-90 percent of the time, consume only whole, organic vegetables, fruits, and meats. Eat locally as much as possible, and in season. Remember to keep alcohol intake to a minimum (or none at all). Remove all controversial foods (processed foods with harmful ingredients.) Eat non-GMO (Genetically Modified Organism) foods. Utilize local, raw honey if tolerated.

Stress—Discern your stress triggers and address them. Find activities you like to do that make you feel alive and empowered. Fit these activities into your schedule and make them a priority.

Breathing—Pay attention to your breathing patterns. When you breathe, do you utilize only the upper part of your chest, or do you take full breaths using your diaphragm? You need to utilize your diaphragm. Utilize the 4/7/8 breathing technique from **Chapter 11, Emergency! I'm Stuck at Full Throttle! Stress.**

Movement—Do you allow your body to move, or do you stay sedentary for most of the day? We are meant to be moving. Our bodies quickly atrophy when they are inactive, causing aches and pains.

Self-care—Try some aromatherapy, a hot bath, light some candles, get a massage, have time with nature, schedule time alone, schedule focused time with loved ones, etc. If you haven't had a medical checkup in a while, go to the doctor.

Meditation / Thoughts—Pay attention to where your mind wanders and begin to listen for encouraging thoughts, as well as those thoughts that are toxic. Get help from a coach or counselor to manage your toxic thoughts and fears. Be OK with the present. Wherever you are, be there.

Environment

Products—replace all with non-toxic, environmentally friendly products.

⊕ Household cleaning
⊕ Personal care
⊕ Air fresheners

Allergens—assess your living environment for,

⊕ Mold
⊕ Dust
⊕ Mites
⊕ Pet Dander

Home Textiles—replace all that have toxic emissions.

⊕ Cooking Pans
⊕ Clothing
⊕ Pillows
⊕ Mattress

Relationships

Assess your relationships and consider distancing yourself from people who do not align with your inner voice.

⊕ Is there someone in your life who always demands that you compromise your own self?
⊕ Is there someone in your life that only supports you when there is something in it for them?

- ⊕ Is there someone in your life who purposely harms you either with words or physical abuse?
- ⊕ Is there someone in your life who puts you down to make themselves feel better.

Assessing your relationships and clearing those that do you harm will be scary and may feel very uncomfortable. Once the relationship is gone, you may feel empty, stressed, and confused. Although it was not a healthy relationship, it was most likely a relationship that was important in your life. You may also feel empty when you realize the familiar anxiety you held in your stomach (due to this relationship) is gone. Although this is healthy, it may feel very unsettling.

Detoxification of harmful relationships makes room for positive and supportive relationships, behaviors, and experiences to enter your life.

The prior paragraph regarding detoxing bad relationships also applies to your food. Remember how everything is connected? Let's go ahead and replace the word "relationship" and "relationships" with the word "food" or "foods."

Assessing your foods and clearing those that do you harm will be scary and may feel very uncomfortable. Once the food is gone, you may feel empty, stressed, and confused. Although it was not a healthy food, it was most likely a food that was important in your life. You may also feel empty when you realize the familiar anxiety you held in your stomach (due to this food) is gone. Although this is healthy, it may feel very unsettling.

Detoxification of harmful food makes room for positive and supportive food, behaviors, and experiences to enter your life.

Lastly

Do you recall the symptoms of toxicity we mentioned earlier? Here they are again. Circle any that you recognize yourself having. As you do this, do you notice some redundancy from other chapters? What about your assessment questionnaire? If yes, that is wonderful! You see, everything is connected! The body is an ecosystem, and several things can cause specific symptoms. We must be open-minded and look for all the possible causes of our symptoms.

- Feeling tired even after getting enough sleep
- Cravings
- Feeling hungry all the time
- Strong body odor
- Headaches
- Frequent colds, infections or viruses
- Constipation
- Allergies or hay fever
- Congestion
- Feeling bloated after eating
- Those few extra pounds you can't lose with diet and exercise
- Puffiness
- Itchy skin
- Pain or stiffness in your joints or muscles
- Restless sleep
- Low moods or a foggy mind
- Difficulty concentrating
- Feeling excessively tired and apathetic
- Moodiness and bursts of irrational anger and frustration

Your Personal Journal With Food

Week Number:_____ Date:_____

What did you eat this week?

_____

_____

_____

_____

_____

How many glasses of plain water per day?_____
What did you do this week that makes you happy?

_____

_____

Percentage of processed foods this week:_____

Percentage of Mindful meals this week:_____

Better Performance Tracker

	Mon	Tue	Wed	Thu	Fri	Sat	Sun
Physical Activity							

CHAPTER 10

An Important Detour—
The Controversies of Food
By Tracy and Ingrid

As you continue your personal journey, one road you must take will be filled with controversy. When you travel this road, you will discover how you personally fit into the "industry" of food. You will find good things as well as things that are apt to be very frustrating. As you become clear about your position in the food industry, you will become empowered and more confident in the decisions you make about your food. The "Road of Controversy" will help you begin considering how your food is processed, packaged, and sold to you. It will enable you to gain the insight needed to make the right choices of food for you and your family.

Over the past 60 years, our food (and its supply chain) has dramatically changed. Humans continue to distance themselves more and more from "real" food. Do we understand what "real" food is anymore? As we continue to distance ourselves from "real" food, we continue to solidify the relationship with what we think food is. This relationship with "food-like substances" makes us believe we don't need to consume anything else. This relationship with "fake" food is not healthy.

It is a mindless and disrespectful relationship with ourselves and our environment. As I discuss in **Chapter 5, Time for an Alignment—The Path of Mindfulness**, we carelessly put "food" into our mouths. We don't ask ourselves these important questions; "By eating what is on my plate, will I be positively serving my body, or am I disrespecting it and setting it up to fail?" "By eating the food I have chosen, am I instructing my cells to produce healthy cells, or am I telling them to produce sick and undernourished cells?"

Wake Up Sleepy Head

I feel as if I have lived in the Matrix all my life, then one day, I literally woke up. I had the choice to take the Blue Pill or the Red Pill. I chose the red pill. I wanted to wake up and get control of my health and my life. For those not familiar with the Matrix, or the concept of the "Red Pill vs. the Blue Pill," Wikipedia explains; *"The red pill and its opposite the blue pill are popular culture symbols representing the choice between embracing the sometimes painful truth of reality (red pill) and the blissful ignorance of illusion (blue pill)." The terms, popularized in science-fiction culture, are derived from the 1999 film The Matrix. In the film, the main character, Neo, is offered the choice between a red pill and a blue pill. The blue pill would allow him to remain in the fabricated reality of the Matrix, therefore, living the "ignorance of illusion" while the red pill would lead to his escape from the Matrix and into the real world. Therefore, living the "truth of reality" even though it is a harsher more difficult life.*

The result of choosing the "Red Pill" was significant for me. I now see the actual reality of our world's food industry. I no longer see it through the eyes of blind, blissful ignorance. Once I woke up, I had the opportunity to walk a new road, although extremely challenging, and sometimes, laden with failure. This road led me to a place where I feel better than I ever have in my entire life. Being willing to change the way I ate and how I viewed not only my food, but myself was not easy for me, but my desire to improve was great. Because I was willing to change my relationship with food, not only did it help me, but it helped my entire family.

How do I continue to navigate The Road of Controversy? One step at a time! When I first started, I could only focus on one thing at a time. Any more than that was overwhelming, stressful, and made each step I took seem more daunting!

I began to look at my habits around processed food and questioned how they served me. Were they undermining or supporting my health? When I discovered a habit that was not helping me, I had to acknowledge it and find a new, supportive habit to replace it. For example, when I would see the drugstore that carried my favorite candy, I would mindlessly head into the store to get it without questioning my actions. I was an addict. I didn't think about it. I was programmed. Now when I see the drugstore, I still think of the candy at times, but I don't mindlessly go in and purchase it. I think first and decide that saving the time, money, and calories for something else is a much better choice! (Not to mention protecting my body from the assault that would happen to it if I ate the candy.)

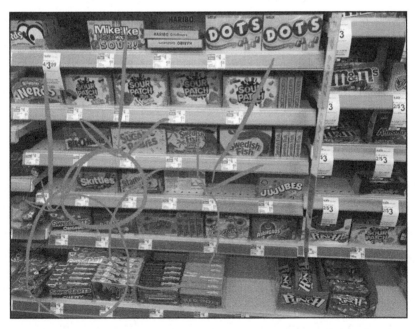

This grocery isle used to OWN me.

This "truth of reality," and understanding the food industry much better, no matter how frustrating it was and sometimes still is, has allowed me to create a healthier relationship with "real" food. Yes, I still have moments where my choices may not be the best, but these are far and few between now. They are not the daily occurrence they once were. I am walking the road. I am stronger. I am continuing to become healthier and happier because of the journey.

What's Your Programming?

It is essential to understand that, as Dr. Mark Hyman states, "Food is Information." Meaning, what you eat causes your body to respond. Will the food you eat help your body balance hormones or send them off on a crazy hormonal up and down rollercoaster ride? Will your food give your body information allowing wellness, or will your food provide information causing illness and disease? Will the food you give your body tell it to burn fat or store fat? How do you get through all the noise? How do you begin to know?

How do you know that your food is giving "good information" to your body and not "bad information?" In **Chapter 6, Your Journey Buddies—Symptoms as a Co-Pilot**, Ingrid discusses the effects of food on our body. Paying attention to these symptoms, however small, and revising your "fuel" intake in response is the best way to know.

Programming is in the Labels

Did you know that the most unhealthy and harmful foods are the most marketed? They have pretty colors on the box, the exciting commercials, etc. So, getting past the marketing and reading all the labels on a product is so important.

One of the best things you can do for your health is to learn how to read food labels. I'm not talking about just the labeling on the front of the product. I'm talking about the nutritional facts section and the ingredients section as well.

When I work with my clients, we discuss food choices. Together we navigate their current diet and consider how it is currently serving them.

As we examine their food choices, we begin to expose the foods that are potentially undermining their ability to feel better, have energy, lose fat, etc. We become "investigators," and we start questioning the validity of nutrition within all the foods they choose to purchase and then eat.

Yes, I understand that label reading isn't the most fun thing to do, let alone the easiest. It was overwhelming for me in the beginning, and I didn't want to have to spend the time learning. I didn't understand how to interpret labels. I also wanted to live in blind bliss. I didn't realize how my lack of knowledge was undermining my health. Fast forward to today; I love reading labels because they immediately help me to know if I should purchase a product or not.

The Misleading Labels of an Industry

We must understand that our food is part of a large global food industry made up of corporations, and like all industries, its purpose is to make money. I don't have a problem with businesses making honest incomes. I do have a problem with companies and industries making money when they know they are manufacturing, selling, and marketing harmful products, yet making it difficult for a consumer to understand this due to their misleading marketing and misleading packaging.

Be sure to look past the commercials and front labels of products. Just because the commercial or the front label says any of the following doesn't mean it will be nourishing for your body.

100% Nutrition, Wholesome, The Best Start for Your Day, Organic, Includes Essential Vitamins and Minerals, Gluten-Free, Natural, Sugar-Free, Whole Grain, etc.

The first things I read when I turn over a package of food, are sugar and salt content, serving size, and then the list of ingredients.

Breakfast Cereals

These don't even get into my shopping cart anymore. When I think back regarding how I started not only my day with cereal but my children's, I realize why we all the symptoms we had. Remember, I didn't understand labels at the time. I believed the front of the box.

Serving Size:

Most cereals today have serving sizes of 3/4 to 1-1/4 cup. I recently did some research on a cereal that was promoted on TV as being very healthy and very nutritious. The serving size was 1 cup. (To help you visualize this, please go to your kitchen and get a 1 cup measuring cup.)

When I looked at the sugar content of this cereal, it was 11 grams. (There are 4.2 grams in one teaspoon of sugar, but nutrition facts round down to 4.0, so keep that in mind as you read labels.) There were approximately 2.62 teaspoons of sugar in a one-cup serving of this cereal.

Now, get out your measuring spoons and measure 2.62 teaspoons of sugar into the cup. Being able to see how much sugar is in this one-cup serving, what are your thoughts?

Now, let's look at the ingredients list of this cereal. Ingredients are listed in order of the highest quantity, to least.

Do you see any concerning ingredients?

1) WHOLE GRAIN OATS, 2) WHOLE GRAIN WHEAT, 3) SUGAR, 4) CORN SYRUP, 5) BARLEY MALT EXTRACT, 6) BROWN SUGAR SYRUP, 7) WHEAT FLAKES, 8) MALT SYRUP, 9) RICE FLOUR, 10) SALT, 11) OAT FLOUR, 12) WHOLE GRAIN RICE, 13) CANOLA OIL, 14) NATURAL AND ARTIFICIAL FLAVOR, 15) RED 40, 16) BLUE 2 AND 17) OTHER COLOR ADDED, 18) SOYBEAN AND CORN OIL, 19) SUCRALOSE, 20) MOLASSES, 21) HONEY, 22) CORN STARCH, 23) ALMOND FLOUR, 24) NONFAT MILK, 25) VITAMIN E (MIXED TOCOPHEROLS) AND 26) BHT ADDED TO PRESERVE FRESHNESS. (BHT is added to keep vegetable oils from going rancid.)

Notice that the 3rd ingredient is sugar, the 4th is corn syrup, the 6th is brown sugar syrup, the 8th is malt syrup, the 19th is sucralose, the 20th is molasses, and the 21st is honey. ALL of these ingredients are a form of SUGAR. Sugar is hidden in most processed, packaged foods. Of the 26 ingredients in this cereal, SEVEN of them are some form of sugar!

Ingredient #13 is Canola oil. Canola is a controversial oil and stands for Canadian Oil. Today, most of the world's canola crop has been genetically altered. It's manufacturers market it as the healthiest option regarding oil. Canola Oil manufacturers call it the "world's healthiest cooking oil!" But is it? Canola oil is processed using extremely high heat and with a toxic solvent called hexane that is used to extract the oil from the seed. Please do some research on this ingredient. Learn how it is made. Once you've done this, are you sure you want to put this ingredient into your body?

Now, let's take a look at the rest of the ingredients listed on the label.

Ingredient #14: Natural and Artificial Flavor. This is the only information we receive regarding flavors added to the cereal. Hmmm, what are they? We are not able to learn this from the label. Personally, I want to know what the artificial and natural flavors are!

Ingredients #15, 16 and 17: Red 40, Blue 2, and "other color" added. What are these ingredients, and how do they impact my body? You must do your research. Food colorings such as Red 40 and Blue 2 have been linked to cancer, hyperactivity, allergies, etc. A simple website that has put together some excellent information and resources about food dyes is https://www.special-education-degree. net/food-dyes/.

Remember, this box of cereal advertised itself as a very healthy way to start your day. One thing I hadn't stated yet was that the front of the box led me to believe there were blueberries and pomegranate in the cereal. I did not find any blueberries or pomegranates listed anywhere in the ingredients list.

Below are some questions I asked myself when I read the information on the label:

How can this cereal be a healthy way to start the day when just one 1-cup serving contains 2.62 teaspoons of sugar, controversial food colorings, and oils? What is this company's definition of healthy? I can see it is different than mine.

Will people have just one serving at a time? In my workshop "How to Let Go of the Yo-Yo, Why Diets Don't Work," attendees are asked to pour themselves a bowl of cereal. Inadvertently, they pour well over the allotted serving amount into their bowls. Many poured upwards of three to 4 times into their bowl. They did this because they didn't believe that a 1 cup serving would be enough to keep them feeling satisfied and full. Now I think about the person who poured three to four 1 cup servings into their bowl and unknowingly ingested nearly eight teaspoons or more of sugar for breakfast!

Next, I think about the children served this healthy cereal every morning. I put myself in the place of a parent who believes they are starting their child out with a wholesome breakfast. But inadvertently send their child to school with upwards of 8.25 teaspoons of sugar, food colorings, and other questionable ingredients flooding their bloodstream. (I did this!) This is happening day after day, and we wonder what is wrong with our children? We wonder why they are agitated, anxious, and why they can't concentrate in school.

Three servings of this cereal contain 33 grams of sugar. (Remember how the nutrition facts round down by .2 grams? So, in actuality, three servings contain 33.6 grams.) The American Heart Association recommends the maximum amount of added sugar to be consumed by a man per day is 36 grams, 25 grams for women, and 25 grams for children between the ages of 2 and 18

Ready for a Warm Bowl of Soup?

Cereal is just one area where marketing and front labels can be misleading to the consumer. Soups and broths are also culprits. It doesn't matter if the front label says organic, all-natural, wholesome, warm goodness, etc. It doesn't matter if the soup is packaged in a can or a box. Turn that package around and read the ingredients and the nutritional facts. Be sure you know if the container is one serving or more. Then look immediately for the sodium content as I find this to be the biggest issue with soups and broths. I will see upwards of 1000+ mg of sodium in a single one-cup serving. Some cans or boxes of soup include what is considered two servings. If you eat a complete can or box of soup, you could be unknowingly consuming 2000+ mg of sodium in just one meal. The American Heart Association is recommending that adults be at no more than 1500 mg of salt per day. Do you want to ingest all of your sodium in a one-cup serving of soup?

Here are some helpful articles regarding sodium:

FDA: https://www.fda.gov/food/nutrition-education-resources-materials/use-nutrition-facts-label-reduce-your-intake-sodium-your-diet

The American Heart Association: https://www.heart.org/en/healthy-living/healthy-eating/eat-smart/sodium/how-much-sodium-should-i-eat-per-day

Food Across the Continents

HEINZ KETCHUP
Canadian Ingredients
Tomato paste made from fresh ripe tomatoes, liquid sugar, white vinegar, salt, onion powder, and spices.

US Ingredients
Tomato concentrate, distilled vinegar, high fructose corn syrup, salt, spice, onion powder, natural flavoring.

UK Ingredients
Spirit vinegar, sugar, salt, spice and herb extracts (contains celery), spice (Interesting that there is no tomato listed in the UK ingredients list.)

RITZ CRACKERS
Canadian Ingredients

Enriched wheat flour, soybean oil, cheddar cheese (milk ingredients, bacterial culture, salt, microbial enzyme, calcium chloride, colour, lipase), sugar, salt, baking soda, malted barley flour, calcium phosphate, spices, ammonium bicarbonate, colour (contains tartrazine), protease, amylase.

US Ingredients

Unbleached enriched flour (wheat flour, niacin, reduced iron, thiamine mononitrate, riboflavin, folic acid), whole grain wheat flour, soybean oil, sugar, partially hydrogenated cottonseed oil, leavening (calcium phosphate, and/or baking soda), salt, high fructose corn syrup, soy lecithin.

UK Ingredients

Wheat flour, vegetable oil, sugar, raising agents (ammonium and sodium bicarbonates, disodium diphosphate), salt, glucose syrup, barley malt flour.

What are your thoughts about the ingredients in the Ritz crackers made in the United States vs. the other countries? Why do you think the ingredients are different for each country?

Let's hear from Ingrid regarding labels in her home country, Chile.

Chilean Labels

As in the United States, the people of Chile are also confused as to what is and is not considered a healthy food.

In 2016, the government of Chile began regulating the labeling of national products. The government has a compelling reason to do so: Chile has the highest rate of adult obesity in Latin America. And the percentage of overweight and obese children has doubled in ten years, which means that five out of 10 kids are overweight or obese. This has sparked an alarming increase in type II diabetes (and other diseases related to obesity) in children.

The solution proposed by the government was to review food labeling and, according to nutritional criteria, alert the public to products that are high in FAT, CALORIES, SUGAR, and SODIUM per individual serving.

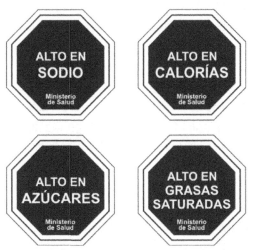

Photo source: Chilean Ministry of Health

As a result, every product manufactured in Chile, that is high in fat, sugar, sodium, or calories has a black stop-sign shaped label placed on the packaging to alert consumers.

It is a good start. It is helping people learn to be more mindful about what they are consuming, but in reality, it is not an educational tool because:

1. There is no discrimination between good and bad fats.

You see, your body needs fat; omega 3 and omega 6 in the proper amounts, for example. However, in Chile, you will see a big black stop sign on a package of healthy raw cashews. The same label you will find on a package of fries loaded with trans-fats, which are very unhealthy fats.

2. The same issue with CALORIES.

There is a big difference in calorie QUANTITY and calorie QUALITY. An average person will need about 2000 calories per day to live. Know that not all calories are equal, however!

In Chile, there is a belief that fewer calories are always better. But we have to realize that a zero-calorie diet soda, loaded with chemicals, cannot be a better choice than a 94 calorie, nutrient-rich green juice! How about we reduce the poor-quality calories from our diets and increase our nutrient-dense calories?

3. It is based on serving sizes:

In Chile, the food industry reacted very quickly and revised its packaging to eliminate the "Stop Sign" requirements on their products. How did they do this? By reducing the size of the package and quantity of "food" in each package, they were able to sell and market the same unhealthy product as a healthy product. Even though it is still loaded with sugar, high sodium, and unhealthy fats. All because they were able to get around the stop sign labeling.

4. The packaging doesn't alert you to controversial ingredients.

Ingredients like preservatives, artificial colorings, and other chemicals the industry may add to food are not listed. These ingredients could be a risk to your health if consumed.

5. It demonizes all food with stop-signs, healthy or not.

People may think that a "Sign Free" product is healthy even when it is loaded with chemicals. For example, diet products with chemical sweeteners that are linked to cancer may not have a "Stop-Sign."

So, the solution is to recognize what real nutrition is. Consume label-free whole foods such as fruits, vegetables, whole grains, legumes, and good quality meat if you eat meat.

There are many other essential things Ingrid and I would like to go over in this chapter, but we will have to keep those for another book. In the meantime, you can research the following:

- ⊕ Grass-fed meats vs. feed-lot meats
- ⊕ Organically grown produce vs. conventionally grown produce
- ⊕ Genetically modified organisms and their implications not only on our health but the health of bees, other insects, and worms.
- ⊕ Enzyme additives
- ⊕ Palm oil
- ⊕ Fructose and High Fructose Corn Syrup
- ⊕ Food colorings
- ⊕ Anything else that you see on a label that you are not fully understanding

Conclusion

We all must understand, we are consumers, and like all consumers, our purpose is to purchase what the food industry and corporations sell. Or is it? Think about this for a minute. We have been programmed to think we need all these processed foods. Do we honestly need all these options? Do we need to continue to participate as you have been? We do not.

The good news is you can participate as an educated consumer. You can choose right now to take the "Red Pill," as I did, and wake up. Join me and start making informed decisions immediately when it comes to what you are going to allow your hard-earned dollars to purchase. Join me and start making mindful decisions as to what you are going to allow into your priceless body.

Life is challenging enough. Stress and anxiety, due to everyday living, is amplified when the wrong food is given to our body's cells. I found that the ingredients in the foods I used to eat not only caused me great physical and mental distress but that these foods also caused distress to many others. The distress I speak of is to our own personal health as well as to our global ecosystem. With that said, different regions of the world have different food available to them. Wherever you live, do your best with what food is available. Can you seek out other grocery stores/food delivery options to help you get the healthiest food possible?

Being healthy shouldn't have to be hard. Food shouldn't be difficult, but it HAS become difficult. Make the empowering choice to be knowledgeable about your food.

The following exercise will help you become wise to the marketing tactics of food corporations and will help you discern what foods you are willing to purchase and then eat. Remember, our food is absorbed, thus becomes our body.

Exercise: Question and Investigate

Ask questions and be an informed consumer by doing the following:

⊕ Begin to question all food product marketing you see. For example, if you see a commercial promoting a "healthy" cereal, yogurt, or weight loss product, take a moment to go to your computer and research the nutritional facts and the ingredients of that product. Are all the ingredients easily understood, or do you see a mystery word or words listed? If there are mystery words, take a moment to look up what they are so you can make an educated decision.

⊕ Grocery Store Tour: Do some investigative reporting. Have fun with this and involve your friends, family members, and your children. Be investigators as you tour the various food aisles of the store.

- Take note of all the following:
- Where are all the food products located?
- The actual serving size of any product and determine what that looks like physically.
- The nutritional facts list, i.e., how much sugar? How much sodium/salt? What else do you see?
- The ingredients list: How many ingredients are there? What are the first five ingredients? Are there any mystery ingredients? What else do you notice?

- Take note of products that are specifically marketed to children. For example, these could be cereals, frozen foods, yogurts, cheese, juices, candy, lunch meats. Where are these products located in the store? What are their ingredients?

- Dairy section: Milk, creamers (whole dairy, fat-free dairy and non-dairy), yogurt, etc. Compare them to each other. What differences do you see in the ingredients of the whole milk, 2% milk, or fat-free milk? What do you think is the better choice to make? Compare the yogurt. Can you find any that do not have a high level of sugar? Can you tell if any of the sugar is added or a natural part of the original "whole" food?

- Frozen Food section: Pizzas, pre-made diet entrées, ice-cream.

- Health Food section: Dairy, cereals, bread, etc. (Tip: just because an item is in the Health Food section, doesn't mean it's healthy.)

- Bread aisle: white, wheat, whole grain bread, hot dog, and hamburger buns.

- Soups and Sauces aisle: spaghetti, pizza, Alfredo, Asian, Mexican.

- Meats: Fresh and frozen beef, poultry, seafood.

- Is there anything else you can think of that you may want to review at the store?

- Shop mindfully and ask these questions:

  "Will this product nourish?"

  "Will this product cause harm?"

  "Am I willing to put this product in my own body?"

  "Do I feel confident serving this to my loved ones?"

  "How can I provide a healthy alternative if the

choice I am looking at does not provide REAL nutritional value?"

"How can I start integrating healthier options into my life? For example, maybe I don't like the taste of the healthier ketchup option, but maybe I can combine my favorite ketchup with the healthier ketchup in the meantime. Over time, I can transition my taste-buds to the healthier ketchup option. I could do this with many of the food items I buy!"

⊕ Home Tour: Utilize the same skills you learned in your Grocery Store Tour and inspect all the food you have in your own pantry, refrigerator, and cupboards. What do you see? How many products will you replace? See if you can find products with less sugar, sodium, and additives.

Overall, just do your best. You may find that one of your favorite products is not what you thought it was. This can be really disappointing. Just be prepared for this to happen. If it does, it's ok to be frustrated and a bit sad. Begin putting your mind to finding an alternative.

Your independent journey on the "Road of Controversy" starts here. Congratulations, you are now better able to discern products that might appear to be healthy but aren't necessarily healthy for you! We hope you will continue to use what you've learned and continue to investigate even further. Now that you are armed with the knowledge outlined in this chapter, the next time you go to the store to make a food purchase, you will have the ability to make mindful choices that will better serve your body.

Your Personal Journal With Food

Week Number:_____   Date:_____

What did you eat this week?

_____

_____

_____

_____

_____

How many glasses of plain water per day?_____
What did you do this week that makes you happy?

_____

_____

Percentage of processed foods this week:_____

Percentage of Mindful meals this week:_____

Better Performance Tracker

	Mon	Tue	Wed	Thu	Fri	Sat	Sun
Physical Activity							

After your pantry tour: How many products will you replace for others with fewer ingredients or with less sugar, sodium, and additives?

_____

_____

_____

CHAPTER 11

Emergency! I'm Stuck at Full Throttle! Stress

By Tracy

What does stress have to do with food? A great deal!

There are different types of stress. Some stress is good for us, but not all. How do you know if you are experiencing good stress or bad?

Good (useful) stressors are those that are intermittent. Our body goes into stress mode to get you out of danger. Consider your car; you have to throttle quickly or break quickly to keep it out of danger, but you don't drive that way all the time because it would cause you to burn too much gas and to go through brake pads very quickly! Your body is the same; sometimes you have to make a quick decision to speed up, run, or stop to stay safe. Another way you may experience stress is if you are trying something new and are feeling nervous for a brief period. In both these examples, the stress leaves you after the incident is over, and your body settles back down.

Chronic stress is a persistent, on-going, long-term situation. Chronic stress is very harmful, and it is damaging to the mind and body. Dr. Mark Hyman, founder and medical director of The UltraWellness Center, states that 95% of all illness is either caused by or worsened by stress. A damaged immune system, leaky gut, weight gain, insulin resistance, pre-diabetes, damaged brain cells, chronic inflammation, sleep impairment, triggering autoimmune disorders, and common viruses and flu, to name a few, can all be linked to stress.

Stress is not meant to be persistent, on-going, or long term. It's intended to turn on for a short period, then to shut off again. Chronic stress in the body is like a car in which the accelerator does not ease up. If not corrected, the car will run out of gas or lose control and crash.

When your body is under constant stress, cells are forced to perform long-term in ways they were only meant to perform for in short periods. They do not function properly. Under this duress, you would most likely experience symptoms as noted above as well as overeating, under-eating, cravings, weight loss, weight gain and gut problems (to name a few), all resulting in damage to body organs over time. And stress can cause a great deal of harm to a person emotionally, as well as to others around them.

I didn't realize I had chronic stress. Not only did I not know what it was, but I was also in denial about stress overall. I was ashamed of myself when I realized I was so distressed. I placed judgment on myself and was so disappointed that I was not able to handle everything in my life. How weak could I be?

Taking an assessment of your life is extremely important. It can be challenging to look at the reality of things, but until you do, making positive steps to change can't happen. In our **Introduction**, you were able to complete your **Life Radar** circle. If your radar is out of sync, this can cause stress. If you haven't had the opportunity to complete your **Life Radar**, go back to the **Introduction** and do so now before going any further.

Our society demands that we participate in its fast-paced, multi-tasking, information-overloaded environment. When I try to explain the way I feel in this environment, I parallel it to how I would imagine hundreds of little gnats and flies annoying me, biting at me and distracting me at every turn. The day I realized I do not have to participate and accommodate the "demands" of this noisy society, my stress dropped immensely.

Realize you are not weak because you cannot handle EVERYTHING.

Stay in the present moment. Focus on one thing at a time. Multi-tasking does not work because it confuses the brain. Our brains can only focus on one thing at a time. Be mindful of where you are and what you are doing. Minimizing stress does not have to be complicated.

Take some time to write down all your concerns. Find a friend or a coach to go over them with you and help you prioritize them. Find the top three priorities. Delegate the next group, if at all possible, and just let go of the rest. (Regarding delegating, you must learn this skill. There are people out there that can do the things you need to have done. Find someone to help and just let go.)

Breathing

You can start with one of my absolute favorite breathing techniques. I learned this from Dr. Weil, of the Arizona Integrative School of Medicine.

If you find yourself feeling distressed, utilize the following breathing technique to reset your body to a calm state:

- ⊕ Relax your shoulders and mouth
- ⊕ Focus on your breathing. Is your breathing shallow (only in the upper portion of your chest), or are you breathing deeply, down into your diaphragm and lower abdomen? If you are breathing, shallow, see if you can start moving that breath deeper into your abdomen and diaphragm. Once you have done this, do the following:
- ⊕ Breath in through your nose for the count of 4
- ⊕ Hold for the count of 7
- ⊕ Release through your mouth for the count of 8

You can do this technique at any time; no one has to know. Try this exercise while; driving in traffic, sitting in a stressful meeting at work, at your desk, just before making a speech or presentation, or just before having a discussion with your child regarding their behavior.

Dr. Weil recommends that you do this exercise every morning before you get out of bed, at midday, and just as you are getting into bed to go to sleep. If you do this, you will start to see not only that your stress levels have lowered, but your body will start showing signs of improvement in many other ways.

Physical Exercise

Exercise is a phenomenal stress reliever. Our bodies were not meant to be kept stagnant. They need to be moving, so it is essential to allow your body to move. Set a timer to remind yourself to get up and move during the day. I recommend setting a reminder for every 40 minutes. Get up from your desk and stretch, take a walk down the hall, breathe nice and deep, then smile! Congratulate yourself on allowing yourself this moment! Commit to moving.

Mindfulness and Meditation

As I write in **Chapter 5, Time for an Alignment—The Path of Mindfulness**, by staying present and keeping your mind in the present moment, allows for calmness. Breathing, as Dr. Weil teaches, then bringing your focus on to one thing helps the mind calm down, brings down your heart rate as well as adrenaline and cortisol levels.

Awareness is the key. Be aware of your stress triggers and catch yourself when you begin to feel stressed. Be sure to breathe. Awareness is half the battle. When you are aware, you can do something about it.

Isolation

Isolation from the hectic aspects of life can be very good and necessary but be aware if you find yourself isolating yourself more and more. Interacting with others is a crucial part of being human. We are social beings. Chronic isolation can cause stress to the body and loneliness. If you find yourself in a position of isolation, do your best to "step out into the world." Find your tribe and make connections that warm your heart and soul. If you aren't sure where to start, consider volunteering for your community. When we give, we actually gain far more than we could have ever imagined.

Prioritize

Be realistic about what you can accomplish in a day. I had to spend a great deal of time on this. Being a bit of an overachiever, I wasn't realistic with myself about what I could achieve in one day. This mindset caused me loads of unnecessary stress.

Plan ahead. Plan time for breakfast, lunch, and dinner and put them on your calendar. Be sure to include the preparation time for each meal. Plan time for exercise and make it a priority. Plan time to breathe and get centered.

Take the time that you've dedicated to habits that don't serve you and give that time to self-care. You might believe that taking care of your own needs is selfish. The fact is, if you don't take care of yourself, you won't be able to stay healthy physically and emotionally. And if you don't take care of yourself, you probably won't be able to take care of those you love when they need you.

Being creative and looking at ways to de-stress your life is essential and a priority for a healthy life.

Take a moment now to list all the things that are bringing stress into your life. Again, there is no judgment here. Just list them.

Now, put your mind to the task of prioritizing them in order of the highest stressor to lowest. When you're finished, look at the list and see which of these stressors can be deleted because they aren't a priority at this time. Let them go. It may be hard, but letting go can feel sooooo good!

If one of the tasks on your list cannot be removed, can you delegate it to someone else? (Don't be superhero here and tell me you can't delegate. You can.)

Do you need to seek professional help or advice to handle some of these stressors? There's no shame in asking for help. Asking for help does not mean you're a failure. Asking for help is an act of courage.

Again, put your mind to the task of solving your stress challenges. See if you can agree with yourself on what your top three priorities are. Everything else can be set aside or delegated.

Write down your top three priorities here. (I'm hoping that one of these top three priorities relates to taking care of you.)

_____

_____

_____

Now, commit to these three items.

Commit to finding others to whom you can delegate.

Your Personal Journal With Food

Week Number:_____ Date:_____

What did you eat this week?

_____

_____

_____

_____

_____

How many glasses of plain water per day?_____
What did you do this week that makes you happy?

_____

_____

Percentage of processed foods this week:_____

Percentage of Mindful meals this week:_____

Better Performance Tracker

	Mon	Tue	Wed	Thu	Fri	Sat	Sun
Physical Activity							
478 Breathing							
Top 3 Priority Task							

CHAPTER 12

Rest Stop—Time to Get Some Much-Needed Sleep
By Tracy

In today's busy, multi-tasking, wired world, it can be challenging to slow down to let the body fully rest. It seems that many people, myself included at one time in my life, feel that they MUST sacrifice sleep. They pride themselves on getting minimal sleep.

"Sleep is for the weak."

"There's no time to sleep. When you die, you will sleep enough."

These are just a few of the things I have heard people say in the past.

This attitude towards sleep is causing many people a great deal of distress mentally and physically.

What happens when you don't get enough sleep? Here is a list of symptoms related to sleep deficiency.

- Sugar cravings—The brain needs the energy to stay awake; therefore, lack of sleep increases cravings.
- Weight gain
- Appetite regulation hindered

- Emotional tolerance is low. Mood swings are more common.
- Intelligence drops
- Forgetfulness
- Impaired judgment
- Confusion and poor concentration
- Trouble being alert
- Ability to make decisions is compromised
- Productivity drops
- The ability for the body to detox, compromised
- Cell regeneration, compromised
- Insulin resistance, even in those that are not obese
- Increased stress levels
- Disruption of the immune system—more apt to get sick from viruses and bacteria
- Disruption of gut bacteria—more susceptible to Leaky Gut Syndrome
- Harms brain, disrupting neurotransmitters
- Mitochondrial function hindered
- Central nervous system impaired
- Reaction time impaired
- Endurance and energy capacity are impaired
- Motivation to exercise is reduced
- Increased risk of heart disease
- Increased risk of Inflammatory illnesses

Benefits of Sleep
The opposite of all the above.

Burning the Midnight Oil
For us to be able to "burn the midnight oil," we have to continue to feed our brain. The brain is very demanding of our energy intake from foods.

It gets first rights to them. When we stay up late, we are fighting the brains' desire to sleep. It's going to demand that we feed it. Hence, we get the urge to snack, and usually, the desire is to snack on sugary things. The brain loves sugar. It needs sugar to survive. When we burn the midnight oil, we will inadvertently consume more energy (calories) than we would if we just went to bed when we were tired. Thus, we gain weight.

Detoxification

As Ingrid stated in **Chapter 9, Tune-Up—Time to Detox**, we have what is called our circadian rhythm. We naturally ebb and tide with the light and darkness of the day. She stated that when we eat consistently and don't allow for the digestive system to rest, we can cause distress to our body. If we don't sleep long enough, or well enough, our bodies cannot get through the complete detoxification process, thus leaving us feeling tired and flu-like in the morning.

Chronic Sleep Deficit Disorder

I read an article by Vatsal G. Thackee, in the New York Times, from April 27, 2013. In this article, Thackee explains that a chronic sleep deficit can create symptoms that can lead to misdiagnosis of A.D.H.D. (Attention-Deficit Hyperactivity Disorder.)

"Many theories are thrown around to explain the rise in the diagnosis and treatment of A.D.H.D. in children and adults. According to the Centers for Disease Control and Prevention, 11 percent of school-age children have now received a diagnosis of the condition. I don't doubt that many people do have A.D.H.D.; I regularly diagnose and treat it in adults. But what if a substantial proportion of cases are sleep disorders in disguise? For some people—especially children—sleep deprivation does not necessarily cause lethargy; instead, they become hyperactive and unfocused. Researchers and reporters increasingly see connections between dysfunctional sleep and what looks like A.D.H.D., but those links are taking a long time to be understood by parents and doctors."

I recommend reading the article in its entirety at: https://www.nytimes.com/2013/04/28/opinion/sunday/diagnosing-the-wrong-deficit.html?_r=1

Bedtime Ritual

The fear of missing out can make it hard for the brain to calm down and rest. Because of this, it is essential to establish a bedtime ritual that allows your mind to wind down and relax. A routine that will allow your mind to disconnect from all that it is trying to manage. Keeping a good ritual will help reset hormones. It will also help your body make melatonin. Melatonin helps you fall asleep and stay asleep.

Here are ideas that will help you establish a healthy routine for yourself.

- Set an alarm/reminder on your phone that will chime several hours before your desired bedtime, reminding you to start winding down for the day.
- Eat a smaller meal for dinner and limit your food intake several hours or more before bed. This will allow your body to spend time detoxing and repairing vs. digesting.
- Limit alcohol. Alcohol can disrupt your body's rhythm. You may fall asleep immediately after a few drinks, but alcohol usually leads to late-night heart racing, sweats, and sleepless nights.
- Limit water/liquid intake beginning several hours before bed to help limit nighttime bathroom visits.
- Limit caffeine, especially if sensitive to it. It can stay in your system for 8+ hours or so, thus hindering sleep.
- Place a notebook and pen beside your bed so that you can do a brain dump right before laying your head down. By writing down thoughts that come to mind, the mind knows that you will be able to look at the list and thus remember

to do that specific item. By doing this, you will allow your mind to relax. You can also use this notepad if you ever wake up in the middle of the night with a concern or a brilliant idea you don't want to forget.

⊕ Gratitude—take a moment to give appreciation to those you love and all you have. "Count your blessings instead of sheep." Bing Crosby, White Christmas. Have a gratitude journal beside your bed to list all that you are grateful for.

⊕ Limit all blue light. Blue light disrupts the production of melatonin. Limit the use of cellphones, computers, or TVs within 30 minutes of going to bed. (It would be beneficial to get a blue light filter for your computer screens and phone.) No blue light alarm clocks.

⊕ Record favorite late-night TV shows and watch them during earlier timeframes.

⊕ Read for pleasure. Let the brain relax into a story.

⊕ De-stress by taking a soothing bath or shower, stretch, meditate, practice gratitude, have sex, or go for a nice walk.

⊕ Set room up for sleep. Keep the temperature cool. Try to eliminate clutter. Make it a calming space. Get blackout drapes if exterior lighting is too bright and disrupts sleep.

⊕ Utilize a sun lamp for your alarm.

⊕ Leave phones in other rooms.

⊕ Keep your bedroom a little bit cooler at night.

⊕ If you have external noise around your home, consider getting a "white noise" machine or utilize earplugs.

⊕ Turn off Wi-Fi routers.

⊕ Have pets sleep in their own space, not in your bed.

⊕ Do the 4/7/8 breathing exercise recommended in **Chapter 11—Emergency! I'm Stuck at Full Throttle—Stress**

In the Morning

- Stretch and get up right away.
- Don't snooze your alarm clock.
- Take a moment for gratitude.
- Review any notes you wrote down during the night or before bed.

During the day, especially if you don't get exposure to natural sunlight, utilize a sun lamp. A sun lamp will help you reset your circadian rhythm, thus help you to sleep at night. There are various kinds available: small desktop lamps, floor lamps, and ceiling lamps in which to choose.

Tip, if you have been surviving on minimal sleep and you find it hard to start going to bed at a time which allows you adequate time to sleep, move your bedtime schedule up by just 15-minute increments each week. This won't feel like such a shock and may be more manageable for you to get "buy-in" from your "fear-of-missing-out" mind. If you have been going to bed at 1 am, for example, and getting up at 6 am, start on Sunday night going to bed at 12:45. The next Sunday, go to bed at 12:30 and so on. Within no time, you will be able to get your mind to settle in and be in bed at 10 pm.

Another tip I would like to recommend is this. Instead of burning the midnight oil on your weekdays and trying to catch up on your rest all weekend, thus wasting the days away feeling tired, get your sleep in during the week, and then have a glorious weekend being alert and active! Trust me on this one!

Exercise: Prepare for Sleep

1. Review your current bedtime ritual and then pick a few of the suggestions above to begin implementing.
2. Choose a day that you are going to start your new bedtime ritual and get started.

Your body and mind will LOVE you for this!

Pleasant dreams!

Your Personal Journal With Food

Week Number:_____   Date:_____

What did you eat this week?

_____

_____

_____

_____

_____

How many glasses of plain water per day?_____
What did you do this week that makes you happy?

_____

_____

Percentage of processed foods this week:_____

Percentage of Mindful meals this week:_____

Better Performance Tracker

	Mon	Tue	Wed	Thu	Fri	Sat	Sun
Physical Activity							
478 Breathing							
Top 3 Priority Task							
Hours of Sleep							
Bedtime Ritual							

Is My Vehicle Good Enough?
—Self-Image
By Tracy and Ingrid

Who is that person I see when I look in the rear-view mirror?

As a child, I didn't think about how I looked. Not until 6th grade, and a classmate of mine told me I should wear makeup. I wasn't concerned about my weight until my senior year in high school when I started getting curvy, and it seemed like my breasts got everywhere before I did! I didn't value myself any less than any other person until 6th grade when I realized that my family was struggling financially. When you are young, it can be challenging to see things in context, easy to believe you are the only one that may be struggling. My early beliefs regarding my looks, body, and finances, created the beginning of a very rocky time for me. These beliefs that I developed about myself at a young age remained into my adult life.

Incidents during those times challenged my self-image and confidence. Throughout my junior high, high school, and college years, I battled with my self-worth. I was always forcing myself forward despite what was going on and how I felt about it. I guess I am tenacious if nothing else—a fighter. I felt as if I was always clawing for my dreams and trying to feel like a normal kid. (As an adult, I now know that normal is only a perception. It is what I defined it to be.)

Auditioning for school plays, vocal solos, first chair in band, were ways to force me out there. A way to possibly show others I was worth something. I always did things that scared me because inside, something always spoke to me, saying, "You can do this!" I was successful and enjoyed my time on the stage and in my music. BUT the MINUTE I was out of my element of music and the stage, I was just Tracy again. I was just a teen that was struggling inside and was trying to like myself.

When I did achieve something pretty significant, such as the first chair in the band, the lead in the play or musical, the academic award or scholarship, I discounted that achievement because I did not believe I was worthy of the success. "Soon, it will be discovered that you are a fake, Tracy. They will know that you are afraid. They will all learn that you don't have any money. They will all realize you are fat, your hair is wrong, your clothes aren't good enough, look at those thighs. Honestly, yuck! You don't even have that good of a voice!" Oh, my word! What a nasty little you-know-what lived in my head! I would discount every achievement saying to myself, "It's no big deal. If I could do it, then anyone could do it. I wasn't worth much anyway." I understand now that this is called, Imposter Syndrome and many people have these thoughts.

Because of this "Imposter" mindset, I was a chameleon in relationships with others. I would mold myself into who I thought they wanted me to be. Dropping my dreams and valuing all others more than myself. These chameleon relationships only affirmed what that horrid voice in my head would say. "You aren't worth anything. If you don't change who you really are, you will be ALONE and worth even less! You won't have any friends or a romantic relationship. So, what if you have to settle for less or give up who you are to have relationships. If anyone knew the real you, you wouldn't have anyone. You can't let anyone know who you REALLY are because that person isn't worth anything. Just keep pretending." I wasn't living as my authentic self; therefore, I was letting myself down.

In college, my first roommate allowed another girl to bully me. She let another student into our room to ice my bed. That student also wrote horrible things on my dorm room door criticizing me. The way I looked, dressed, danced, sang, you name it. I had a difficult time not believing the mean things she said. Could she be right? I would ask myself. I did not value myself, and I felt the world coming in on me. I wasn't worthy of my goals and dreams. How did I get a scholarship for my voice anyway? It must have been a pity scholarship. I allowed this bullying student to get into my head and affect my decisions while at school. I admit I still hear her at times. I was living from a fear-based mentality, and I didn't know that I could take full responsibility for my circumstances, that I WAS good enough. Talented enough. Worthy.

I felt alone most of my life because I was afraid to talk about my experiences and fears. Afraid to let my guard down. No one else had these kinds of feelings or thoughts. No one had my experiences. I was the only one feeling this way. I was positive that people who were worth anything, never felt as I did. Oh, how I wish I had just spoken up and trusted. I wish that I had believed that being me was more than enough! That I was always enough, and my circumstances were just circumstances. But, I must forgive myself for not speaking up, as I didn't know how to at the time.

Please know, if you are having any challenges or thoughts that are cruel to your well-being, please talk to someone. Know you are not alone. Through these thoughts and fears, you can move forward into a life filled with self-love, amazing friendships and relationships, and PURPOSE.

Now, in my 50's, I can honestly say that I am here on earth for a purpose. I am here for MY PURPOSE, not someone else's purpose. The journey to find this purpose has been filled with grief, frustration, self-doubt, and a period of depression, BUT also full of happiness, love, and joy. You see, when I look back now, I let my mind also find the fantastic and beautiful things that I experienced growing up, in college, as well as in my adult life. I can see the good things that have happened to me and all the beautiful blessings, large and small.

The individual lessons I have learned from the hard times and good times are all similar. I didn't see the lessons before, but now—as I look back on my journey, each lesson moved me closer and closer to who I am meant to be. Each challenge, failure, and success chiseled me into who I am, and I have come to appreciate the experience, empathy, and the strength that each one has given me. I now know that I am the perfect "me" with all my mistakes and imperfections.

Self-image can be tricky. Rising above the negative views of one's self takes work and practice. Lifting a hundred pounds without ever training for it isn't easy either and could be impossible for some. Plus, you would most likely cause injury if you tried! However, with training and practice every day, you could eventually lift 100lbs. With training and practice, you can learn to be kind to yourself. You can learn to be loving towards yourself. You can learn to be caring and passionate towards yourself. Your self-worth is not given to you by others. Your self-worth is already yours! You do not have to give it away to anyone. You don't have to wait for someone to give it to you. It is yours now!

Below are some of the lessons I have learned.

Life has beautiful, as well as traumatic experiences that shape us.
Life is not a race against others.
Life is to be an experience.
Your life is not intended to be someone else's journey.
Life is intended to be YOUR PERSONAL JOURNEY.
Life is a journey to be savored and appreciated.
We can rise above our circumstances.

Once I let go of the belief that I had to live up to everyone else's expectations of me (actually, my imagined expectations that I thought everyone had for me,) a great deal of stress left my body, and my self-image began to climb. Once I decided not to try to be like someone else. I was able to create MY LIFE! I decided to be brave and begin letting go of the perfectionism I held toward myself and my inability to allow myself to make mistakes without flogging myself for days, months, and yes—years.

I now catch myself when I am placing judgment not only on myself but on others. I do my best to be present and embrace not only myself but embrace others where they are.

"Turn your wounds into wisdom."
OPRAH WINFREY

Find and practice gratitude every day. Look for your blessings; the obvious blessings and the not so obvious ones. Find the triumph in your failures. Find forgiveness in your mistakes.

When I look for my blessings, triumphs, and find forgiveness, I find compassion and love for who I am as a person. I have compassion for the person I was, the one who was lost and depressed. I have compassion for the one who was full of anxiety and doubt. I realize that she was an essential part of my journey. She taught me so much!

Self-image is not only aligned with your thoughts; it is aligned with your food as well. They are connected. Food can make us feel a certain way. It can make us feel vibrant, full of vitality, happy, content. Food can also make us feel distressed, sluggish, unhappy, physically bloated, tired. I know now that food had a great deal to do with my feelings of self-worth.

Please know that there have been several times in my life when I gave up. I was so frustrated with my inability to manage my weight, my food, relationships, as well as my career. I hung it all up and decided not to try anymore. After all, nothing was working anyway. I've learned since then that when I value myself, I am more conscious about what I am willing to put into my body, where I am willing to spend my valuable time, and with who I am willing to spend that time. When I am feeling low self-worth, I am more apt to find comfort with foods that will harm my body.

I learned that I had to be at peace with who I was. At peace with all my failures. At peace with EVERYTHING. Even at peace with the decisions that I sometimes wish I could go back in time and change. Once I did that, my life began to change for the better! I released myself from my self-imposed bondage.

Now, I would like to invite Ingrid to tell you about her struggles with self-image.

When I read Tracy's words, I could see my reflection. Despite the distance and different cultural backgrounds, I also grew up with a poor self-image. Today, I still work to elevate my self-image, giving myself the right to deserve the best, and to love me.

When I was born, I surprised my parents. They were expecting a boy. Although they love me, intuitively, I know they were disappointed. And because I intuitively knew this, I pushed myself too much to be like others, and sometimes, I even wished I was a boy. After I was physically abused at only six years old, I so wanted to be a boy. The image of my body was now shrouded in guilt, shame, and vulnerability. I felt scared and wanted to be invisible. At that point, I started to gain weight.

I have read two perspectives about the emotional function of body fat: one is to form a shield to protect you from damage or danger, and the other is your body saying: please see me. See me with love, look at me with compassion. That is what the body is asking, to take care of your wounds with love and care. It took me many years to be able to speak about this abuse and to start accepting and liking the fact that I was a woman. I had to build my self-image from nothing. I found this to be difficult as I was growing up in Latin society with a macho core, where women make extreme efforts to be "beautiful," and everybody gives too much importance to physical appearance.

I grew up in the 1980s when many television shows were beauty pageants. My uncle collected these pageant videos, and as a kid, I watched them a lot. The winners would get diamonds, trips, cars, and everybody's admiration. I believed they also got love and had a wonderful life. How could it be any other way? They were beautiful winners, after all. The beauty queens set an example for me and created a firm belief in me. I believed beautiful people, without cellulite, and with perfect skin, were better. If I wasn't like them, I was not good enough. People in my surroundings always celebrate that kind of beauty: skinny bodies, always looking pretty and neat. Be feminine, as feminine is only in appearance. I began to learn about diets, aerobics, massages, and many other tips that would allow me to fit into the "beauty queen shape."

Peer pressure is a real thing, and the problem was that I was so sensitive to these kinds of opinions. My belief was, "If only you had a pretty and fit body, you would then be loved." I thought love was a reward, but the truth is, love is a right that belongs to every living being.

What are your thoughts and feelings about your body? Do you love your body as is it?

I started to change my beliefs once I understood that the power to change my mindset was within myself. I had heard the quote: "The power is in you." But I didn't know "how" to access that power.

I've learned that the key to finding this power within is to pay attention. Where does your attention go? If your attention focuses only on the things you don't like about your body, you will never be able to be in love with yourself. It's time to focus on the good things about your body:

- ⊕ Your body has the wisdom to keep you alive.
- ⊕ Your legs can take you to experience adventures, see dream-like places, to dance, and have fun.
- ⊕ Your skin feels the expression of love from a caress.

I could go on, but instead, I would like to invite you to do this exercise.

Stand in front of a mirror and look at yourself as a creature of love.

1. Look at your body and think about how you use your body to experience life. Even better: to enjoy life. Do you like to dance? To sing? To walk? Recognize those parts and send love and gratitude to all those body parts, which allow you to experience happiness in life.

2. Look at all the things you most like about your body. Name all the parts of your body you find beautiful, charming, or interesting. Bear in mind that beautiful is a measurement scale.

3. Look at all the things you don't like about your body. What is it that you don't like? Is it how it looks, or is it how it functions? Does this part help you to experience happiness in one moment of your life? Maybe you don't like the way your arms look right now, but I'm sure you love the way your arms hug the people you appreciate. Perhaps a scar is a reminder of strength, being alive, and how you follow your dreams. Create new ways to measure your body.

4. Finally ask yourself, does your body image improve by healthy eating and movement? If so, why not start right now?

Self-Love is another journey Tracy and I invite you to start today.

Food and Self-Image

"As above, so below; as within, so without."

The above quote is from the book, "Kybalion," a hermetic document from the 1800s about spiritual laws that can be applied to food and self-image as we have been discussing it. Food has an energetic side and is not just calories! Food can elevate your mood or make you feel down, just as your thoughts and actions can. Food, emotions, thoughts, and actions all go hand-in-hand.

If I am struggling with my self-esteem, I will have thoughts justifying my current mental state and actions and search for food that keeps me on that downward spiral. Take a moment and think about the foods most people choose when they are sad or heartbroken. What foods do you think of? Are they full of sugar and high glycemic carbohydrates? Foods that only comfort you at the moment but then leave you right back where you started or feeling even worse. I bet you never see this: staying home alone, sad, wearing pajamas, with hair a mess, a box of Kleenex, and a big bowl of celery! No! What you see is a big bowl of chocolate ice cream!

Of course, some of these emotional states will take some time to heal. You need to express your feelings. And once you decide to take care of yourself, improve your self-image, and build a nurturing relationship with yourself, you can also integrate food to help you with that purpose.

You already know which foods deplete you. Start slowly to add positive, energetic whole foods to every meal. You will feel better; you will have a powerful tool to improve the way you feel about yourself.

Embrace your body. Embrace all its curves and imperfections. Be you with no apology. How about measuring your mind and body in supportive ways?

1. The number of days your body is keeping you alive.
2. The number of places you have visited and loved.
3. The number of people you have loved in your life.
4. The number of laughs. (Laughter is said to be the best medicine!)
5. The number of hugs you give.

You can always add more measures to remind you how unique and special you are!

Exercise: Gratitude

Regarding food. Review what you are eating. Pay attention to foods that elevate your spirit and emotions. Make a list of whole foods that you know energize you and add them to your diet this week.

_____

_____

_____

_____

Regarding gratitude, make a list of 10 things you are grateful for and read it every day for 30 days.

_____

_____

_____

_____

What memory or past behavior are you holding on to that make you feel bad about yourself? How can you turn that experience into a blessing and proactive lesson? How can you use that experience to grow and to help others who have experienced the same? Did you know that when we serve others while being genuine and utilizing our purpose and gifts, we then step into our real selves!?

_____

_____

_____

_____

_____

Your Personal Journal With Food

Week Number:_____ Date:_____

What did you eat this week?

_____

_____

_____

_____

_____

How many glasses of plain water per day?_____
What did you do this week that makes you happy?

_____

_____

Percentage of processed foods this week:_____

Percentage of Mindful meals this week:_____

Better Performance Tracker

	Mon	Tue	Wed	Thu	Fri	Sat	Sun
Physical Activity							
478 Breathing							
Top 3 Priority Task							
Hours of Sleep							

Mark the days you have completed your Gratitude exercise.

	Mon	Tue	Wed	Thu	Fri	Sat	Sun
Week 1							
Week 2							
Week 3							
Week 4							
Week 5							

CHAPTER 14

Respect of Inner Self
By Tracy

"Training and managing my own mind, is the most
important skill I could ever own, in terms of both
my happiness and success."

T. HARV EKER

We all have an inspirational, positive, confident, powerful voice inside of us. The strength of that inner voice drives not only why we do the things we do, but also why we feel a certain way about ourselves.

The voice I am speaking of is your Inner Voice, your true self. This voice speaks to you from your gut. This voice speaks to your heart. This voice is your intuition. This voice is your internal guidance system. Fear, the opinions of others, and negative thoughts can stifle this voice, making you feel insecure, less than worthy, disoriented, unhappy. Are you able to hear this empowering voice speak to you? If not, have you silenced it so much that it barely speaks anymore?

Depending on your beliefs, you may call this voice God, the Universe, your soul, or nothing.

One thing I have learned (and I must say I have learned it the hard way)…. You must LISTEN to that voice. Let it be heard and acknowledge what it has to say. Listen to the voice that says, "Keep Going." The one that asks, "Why not you?" and states, "You are worthy." Shine bright! No matter what! Look in the mirror and tell that amazing person "You are here for a reason. You may not know what that is yet, you may not understand your journey or your future path, but you are here for a reason. You are here for a reason which is much bigger than you. Stand tall and be willing to become the person necessary to live your purpose."

As Ingrid and I discuss in **Chapter 13, Is My Vehicle Good Enough? Self-Image**, your inner voice has everything to do with your self worth. You see, our self-worth is not dependent on our physical being. Our self-worth is not dependent on how much we earn or our past experiences that we carry like a heavy backpack on our backs. Our self-worth is not based on what we may have eaten in hiding when no one was looking. We are worth so much more!

Alongside this empowering inner voice, you most likely have another voice inside of you that likes to remind you of all the things that are wrong with you, that you may have done wrong or not accomplished, etc. This voice can make you feel as if you are less worthy than others. Some people like to call this voice Negative Nellie or Negative Ned. Do you have a name for this voice? I definitely do for mine! But I won't write it here in this book! She can be really nasty, mean-hearted, and despicable! I have decided to treat this voice as a separate person and choose to educate her and help her understand why she is not helping me. I also realize that this part of my mind needs to learn new ways of gaining pleasure, new beliefs, a new way to live. I make sure she understands that when she runs the show, things usually don't work out very well for us.

I have to speak firmly to myself (my mind) when I am leaning towards making a choice that will not serve me, such as:

Living from fear and not pursuing my purpose: "I understand you are just trying to protect me, but living in a shell the rest of my life is not going to do us any good. We have to step out and be vulnerable."

Not getting my workout in: "OK, I know you want to be lazy, but we need to get this 30-minute workout in. Remember how good you feel afterward? Remember how proud you are when you get it done? OK. Let's go do it."

Not getting to bed early enough: "I know you want to watch that additional episode of Friends, but you know how hard it is to wake up, you know how hard it is to think, and you know how stressed you get when you don't get enough sleep. Is it really worth it? No. So let's go to bed. You can watch that episode another time. It will still be there."

Drinking too much: "You've had one glass of wine already. I know you feel terrific right now. But is it worth the second or third glass when you wake up at 2 am with your heart racing, and your temperature up as your body tries to process the alcohol and sugar you forced it to take in? Will it be worth the flu-like feeling you will carry with you the next day? Let's go ahead and switch to some water. Your body is going to thank you!"

Eating the cake that I know will make me feel sick: "Yes, it looks great, and you know that some cakes don't make you feel horrible, but you can't guarantee it. Is eating the cake worth your heart rate racing uncomfortably for the next two to three hours? Is this cake worth making your poor tummy bloat out? I don't think so. Who cares if everyone else is having some, your body will thank you for passing on it!"

We are the results of our choices. Over time, these choices (large or even so small) mold us into who we are and create our environment. When it comes to food, we can make decisions that are better for our bodies or decisions that are harmful. When we make better choices for it, we feel more confident and capable, or we can make choices that make us feel resentment towards ourselves and make us feel anguish. Usually, that anguish comes about because we didn't listen to, or acknowledge what our inner voice was trying to say to us. It said, "You aren't hungry. Go ahead and do something else." We choose to ignore it (then feel terrible later, causing us not to respect ourselves.) Our true guidance says, "I love you—do you hear me?" "Let's find something else to do instead of eating that bag of chips. It's going to be OK. We can do this."

Respecting Yourself and Your Path

Listen to your empowering inner voice. It is always speaking.

Learn to say no when your instinct tells you to: Are you a people pleaser? Many people are and will say yes when they know they should say no. We may go along with the crowd when we are aware that this choice will hurt us. We ignore the voice inside us that speaks to the truth of who we are. When we do this, it erodes our self-confidence. It creates a need for approval by others to make us feel we are worthy. What we need to learn is that only we can make ourselves worthy. Only we can do this, and when we do, we create an unwavering self-confidence. We also create a culture within ourselves that is powerful, confident, and secure.

Honor your word to yourself: Let your soul trust YOU. Just like our relationships with other human beings and animals of this earth, we can build a relationship of trust with ourselves. We NEED this relationship with ourselves to be truly healthy.

Do you say you are going to do something that will support you, then turn around and do the exact opposite? Do you tell your soul that you will finally get your eating under control just to break that promise yet again? Do you procrastinate doing the things you know you need to do in other areas of your life? Things that will, over time, get you closer to where you want to go? As in relationships with others, every time we break a promise, the relationship is stressed and moves a bit more towards a breaking point. As it is in relationships with others, it takes work to keep a solid, trusting relationship with ourselves.

Honor your inner self and do for it what you promise to do. Value yourself enough to treat yourself with respect. Honor the body that carries you every day of life on this planet. As you continue to build a healthy relationship, you will notice that making supportive choices for yourself becomes easier and more comfortable. The side of you that looked for approval from others to make decisions will learn to ease up and allow you to be the driver. That is when the magic happens. Walk your talk. Respect your inner voice. Respect yourself.

Speak to yourself with respect. Would you allow others to speak to you as you speak to yourself? Most likely not. I find that when I talk to and listen to my various inner voices with respect and acknowledge what they are saying, my self-worth climbs. You see, that Negative Ned or Nellie are really there trying to protect us. Although it can be terrible in the way they show it. If we acknowledge the thoughts that are fear-based, acknowledge them, then respond in a loving way back, these thoughts begin to wane, and when they do come up, the emotional toll they have on us is less. For example, "You aren't good enough. You will never lose weight successfully. You've never done it before. We will just be disappointed again." We can reply in a kind, loving, but firm way, "I understand why you feel this way. We haven't learned how to do this yet, but that doesn't mean we can't learn. I would really like to have the opportunity to learn how. I know it may be hard, and I most likely will stumble along the way, but I really want to learn. Will you let me learn?"

By communicating compassionately with yourself, acknowledging your thoughts, and by turning the fearful mind into an ally, you can create a supportive environment within yourself.

As you go into this next exercise, bring compassion with you. Don't be afraid to have the inner dialogue between your inner voices—the courageous, positive side and the fearful, protector side. They are both important to you and your success. Practice speaking with respect when you write your answers. Leave accusations aside, have compassion for who you were and who you are today.

Exercise: Honoring and Listening to Your Inner Self

Describe an experience from the past, when you tried to make a decision that honored you and your inner self, but you chose not to.

_____

_____

_____

_____

_____

Describe how you felt during the process of making the decision not to do the right thing for you. What were your thoughts? What conflicts did you have to overcome?

_____

_____

_____

_____

_____

Describe how you felt afterward.

_____

_____

_____

_____

_____

Go ahead and sit with this feeling for a moment. Make your mind understand the implications of making decisions that are harmful to you. Does your mind want you to feel this way again? Is it worth it? Write down your thoughts.

_____

_____

_____

_____

_____

What challenging experience did you have in the past where you successfully decided to follow through and make a decision that honored you and your inner self?

_____

_____

_____

_____

Describe how you felt during the process of deciding to do the right thing for you. What thoughts were going through your mind? What conflicts did you have to overcome?

_____

_____

_____

_____

How did you feel after this decision?

_____

_____

_____

_____

_____

Go ahead and sit with this feeling for a moment. Do your best to educate your mind and help it understand that although the decision to choose kindness towards you and your body was difficult at the time, the overall benefit(s) for it (and you as a whole person) were and are significant.

What were the benefits of making this choice to be kind and caring to you and your inner self?

_____

_____

_____

_____

_____

What have you learned from this exercise that you can take into your daily life to help you make decisions that will benefit your mind, body, heart, soul, and inner self?

_____

_____

_____

_____

Compliment yourself. It can be anything at all. Give yourself a bunch of compliments. Write them down here. You can choose anything you like! Whatever pops up in your mind. Write it down. Don't censor your inner self. Let it speak kind words. (If your Negative Nellie or Ned wants to come to the party and take over, kindly tell them they aren't needed at the moment, and to do something else. You appreciate them wanting to keep you safe, but right now, you will be fine on your own).

_____

_____

_____

_____

_____

Now, let yourself sit with these compliments for a while. Allow yourself to smile. Allow yourself the right to be worthy of them because the truth is, you are worthy of them.

Exercise: Daily Compliments

Write your compliments below and read them daily. Do this every morning when you wake up and every night when you go to bed. By doing this exercise, you allow your mind the chance to learn how to be kind to you. Challenge yourself to keep adding to this list of compliments. As you learn to give genuine gratitude to you, you will be surprised at the gratitude you can then give to others. And you can give it freely and lovingly.

_____

_____

_____

_____

_____

Give yourself the right to live as your true essence, your true self. When you live in that space, you will allow yourself to grow into the person you genuinely respect, a person you genuinely love.

Your Personal Journal With Food

Week Number:_____   Date:_____

What did you eat this week?

_____

_____

_____

_____

_____

How many glasses of plain water per day?_____
What did you do this week that makes you happy?

_____

_____

Percentage of processed foods this week:_____

Percentage of Mindful meals this week:_____

New ways you can positively measure your body and mind:

_____

_____

_____

_____

_____

Better Performance Tracker

	Mon	Tue	Wed	Thu	Fri	Sat	Sun
Physical Activity							
478 Breathing							
Top 3 Priority Task							
Hours of Sleep							

Mark the days you have completed your Gratitude exercise.

	Mon	Tue	Wed	Thu	Fri	Sat	Sun
Week 1							
Week 2							
Week 3							
Week 4							
Week 5							

CHAPTER 15

Continue Your Personal Journey with Food

By Tracy

It's time to review *Your Personal Journey with Food*. First, we want to congratulate you on making a step most will not take. We want to commend you for taking these powerful first steps! Learning to care for yourself and taking the steps needed to understand who you are in relationship to your food, as well as your relationships with all other integrated aspects of your life, allows for a life filled with health-filled opportunities.

Let's take a moment and recap what you have learned so far: You now know that:

⊕ You are a "whole" being. You are not just an arm, leg, heart, brain, etc.

⊕ All aspects of your life; your health, relationships, spirituality, joy, finances, food, physical fitness, and career are intertwined. If one or more of these areas are out of alignment, this can cause distress and frustration in all areas.

⊕ For many reasons, human beings have an emotional connection with food, which begins long before we even understand what food is.

⊕ There is a way you can break free from Yo-Yo dieting and live a healthy lifestyle that supports your body in a way that eliminates the weight fluctuations of the past.

⊕ Symptoms are a gift from the body, alerting us that either something is wrong or what we are doing is supportive of it. When we take action and begin the search for the actual cause of symptoms, our negative symptoms can go away, and we can continue to support our body in ways that it needs to be supported.

⊕ Your body does become what you eat and absorb. Your food becomes your blood, becomes your cells, becomes you.

⊕ Food is information to your cells. Food is similar to a computer software program. When quality software is installed onto a computer, quality computer function will result. For the body, when quality food goes in, proper cell function results.

⊕ Your self-image is not given to you by others. It is yours to give. By looking at yourself through the lens of gratitude, you will increase the positive view of yourself on a daily basis. Being yourself involves no risk. It is your truth.

⊕ Eating mindfully will help you to lose weight, digest food better, make healthier food choices, and help you to fully enjoy food and wonderful treats even more than you did before! You can also take mindfulness into other areas of your life, thus creating an environment that supports you.

⊕ There are different kinds of stress. Short bursts during times of danger or exciting moments. Or on-going, chronic stress that causes inflammation and chronic illness. You have a few new techniques in your pocket now to help minimize chronic stress.

⊛ Your body MUST MOVE! Sedentary lifestyles and poor diets are causing epidemic levels of chronic illness throughout the world. You now know that you can easily exercise throughout the day, even without any equipment or gym membership!

⊛ Even though a specific food may be designated as healthy, it can be harmful to someone who has a sensitivity or allergy to it. You now have skills to help you discover what foods may be detrimental to your body.

⊛ Reading food labels is extremely important, and you must take responsibility to do this. The front of the food packaging (and the commercial on television) does not tell the complete truth. To benefit your health, you MUST read labels.

⊛ Embracing the "whole" you and listening to your inner voice is paramount. Your inner voice is your GPS.

What other things have you learned that we have not mentioned here? Please list them below:

_____

_____

_____

_____

_____

Next, go back to your assessment at the **Introduction**. Find the **Feet on the Pavement View** questionnaire. Date the column on the right. Then rate how you feel now regarding all these various areas of your life. Do you see any changes? Write down your thoughts here.

_____

_____

———————————————————————————

———————————————————————————

———————————————————————————

Now, go ahead and review your **Life Radar,** which you will also find in the **Introduction.** How do you feel about your original plots? Now, re-plot the radar. What does it look like now? In what areas do you feel more confident? Are there any areas that you feel less confident? Write them down here:

———————————————————————————

———————————————————————————

———————————————————————————

———————————————————————————

———————————————————————————

What areas would you like to continue to work on? Commit to doing so.

———————————————————————————

———————————————————————————

———————————————————————————

———————————————————————————

———————————————————————————

———————————————————————————

———————————————————————————

———————————————————————————

———————————————————————————

In closing;

Make your journey here with us your new starting point to lifelong learning, your unique *Personal Journey with Food*. Continue to seek an understanding of your body and its needs. Know that as life changes, your body and mind may need new foods and nutrients. Be willing to ebb and flow with this as you move forward.

Don't be a stranger! We invite you to visit us at **www.journeywithfood. com** to receive any new pdf handouts and to learn about any new programs that will be coming available to you.

Remember, we are here for you and want you to feel free to reach out!

In Health,
Tracy and Ingrid

About the Authors

TRACY

Being told by her doctor in 2006 that she was pre-diabetic and headed towards a future with Type 2 Diabetes, Tracy had to start making better lifestyle choices. A Yo-Yo dieter most of her life, the news was frustrating but put her on her path to wellness. Today, Tracy is no longer pre-diabetic. She is healthy and strong taking on century bike rides, eating in a way that supports her body, and finally feeling good in her skin.

Tracy's health journey inspired her to go back to school and get trained in both Integrative Health Coaching and Personal Training. She is certified with The Institute for Integrative Nutrition, Precision Nutrition, and the National Academy of Sports Medicine.

Tracy is an international best-selling co-author of One Crazy Broccoli, My Body is Smarter Than My Disease! and What's Left to Eat. To learn more about Tracy's coaching programs, visit www.tracycromwell.com or www.journeywithfood.com

INGRID

Ingrid Lauw (born in Paraguay, South America) began her Personal Journey with Food when she was born, and her mom´s breastfeeding was over. At 18, after being a very picky eater as a child (no veggies or fruit,) she moved to Santiago de Chile to live on her own. After years of fast food, sodas, no exercise, tons of sugar, she had a body composition of 40% fat mass. Her body started to have symptoms with no clear diagnosis. She felt ill most of the time and decided she needed to begin taking better care of herself. She listened to her body, learned to cook and make peace with veggies and fruit. She started to exercise and today is a vibrant mother in her 40's with a happy and healthy child.

She is a Certified Integrative Nutrition Health Coach and International Bestselling co-author of *What's Left to Eat.*